Advance

Midlife Women Rock takes a bold and courageous look at menopause and breaking the taboo and shame around this important phase of life which affects half the population. Breeda's passion and mission shine through in every page, empowering and supporting women to embrace this transition and use it as a time to take back control and enjoy the freedom and wisdom of this second stage of life.

- **Nicki Williams,**
- **Happy Hormones for Life**

Midlife Women Rock will be the handbook for all women going through menopause or indeed for others who wish to learn more about a subject that is rarely discussed in public.

The unique informal style, stories, conversations & interviews enclosed all help separate the myths about menopause from the facts, especially as they are described in such an intimate way. I have such admiration for Breeda in sharing her knowledge and resources with us all. The sooner Ireland rolls out the first ever education & awareness campaign the better – a world first.

- **Josepha Madigan**
- **Minister of State for Special education and inclusion**

Menopause is having a 'moment' – with lots of attention and focus from media in the U.K. But simply drawing attention to a problem isn't the same as solving it and what the millions of women 'suffering' through the many symptoms of menopause want is solutions.

With this book, Breeda has brought together provocative prose AND practical advice. Her aims are to challenge the status quo, break down taboos AND provide support and encouragement for women everywhere. She has succeeded!

Sara Price
Rebellious Optimist and Founder of ACTUALLY.WORLD

Breeda is a campaigner, an academic, a field worker, a mother and a real-life, unairbrushed woman.

She speaks for all of us, through her own experience, with compassion, understanding and above all courage helping to change our 'normal' and make all our lives freer.

Sonya Lennon,
Equality advocate and entrepreneur

Breeda's work has shifted the narrative around menopause for the women in the Midlife Women Rock Cafe community and we are thrilled to know how many more people she will reach through this book. The menopause story is changing and the world needs more people like Breeda stepping fully into their power and sharing the message of the transformative experience that menopause can be. A down-to-earth, well-crafted and essential read.

Sjanie Hugo-Wurlitzer and Alexandra Pope
Authors of Wild Power, Discover the Magic of your Menstrual Cycle and Awaken the Feminine Path to Power

In a world which glamorises youth and in particular young women, the particular needs of middle-aged and older women can be overlooked or pushed to one side. This book is starting an important conversation on menopause which for far too long has been a taboo topic. We must move beyond shame and stigma and normalise these conversations and encourage women to seek advice and support. This book successfully combines evidence-based information with real life testimonies making it an accessible and relatable read.

Orla O'Connor .
Director of the National Women Council of Ireland (NWCI)

Midlife Women Rock

A Menopause Story for a New Generation

Breeda Bermingham

Disclaimer

The information in this book has been compiled by way of general guidance in relation to the topics discussed. It is not a substitute for medical, pharmaceutical, healthcare, or other professional advice on specific circumstances and in specific locations. Before stopping, changing, or starting any medical treatment please contact and discuss with your GP.

All names in case stories have been changed. Practice, laws, and regulations all change, and the reader should obtain up to date professional advice on any such issues. The author and publishers disclaim, as far as the law allows, any liability arising directly or indirectly from the use or misuse of the information contained in this book.

As far as the author is aware the information given is correct and up to date as of August 2021.

"What do we live for, if not to make life less difficult for each other?"

George Eliot

Dedicated to John, Laura, Aly, and Will who light up my life every day.

My wonderful Mom, Mary Ellen, sisters Teresa, Eileen, and Angie and

Nana Mary RIP, a true matriarch.

TABLE OF CONTENTS

ABOUT THE AUTHOR

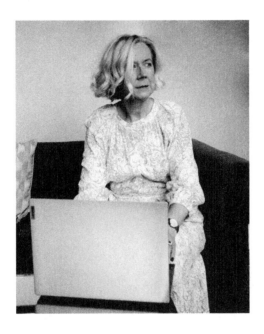

Breeda Bermingham, a menopause advocate and researcher, is the founder of the *Midlife Women Rock Project and Café*. Now a social entrepreneur, she is a former midwife and public health nurse. Following many years working with women in midwifery and in the community in Cork, Dublin, Limerick, and Waterford, she took ten years out of the workplace following the birth of her fourth child. Breeda returned to full-time education at age 49, completing a psychology degree followed by a masters in sociology. During her studies, her interest in menopause was piqued as it aligned with her own experience of this life stage. Having witnessed how essential it is to tackle the taboo and stigma surrounding menopause, supported by Social Entrepreneurs Ireland (SEI), she founded the *Midlife Women Rock Café*. The café allows for the gathering of women in a safe space to talk about menopause while providing information on the stages, symptoms, and management pathways. Working with women in groups and individually, Breeda educates and challenges women's perceptions on negative constructions of menopause witnessing how mindset shifts are a game-changer for so many. *Midlife Women Rock: a Menopause Story for a New Generation* is her first book.

Breeda is available to do podcast guesting, workplace presentations and is a Keynote speaker.

FOREWORD

In a blink of an eye, I find myself in my midlife. The question is, do I still rock in my middle years, or do I fit into the cultural stereotype of invisibility and degeneration? I most certainly do rock, although in a slightly more muted way than in my colourful 20s and 30s. My topic of conversation has now changed from music, parties, and fashion to menopause, HRT, and mental wellbeing.

After discovering a real lack of knowledge around menopause, I have made it my midlife mission to break down the taboo that has shrouded menopause for so many years. I have armed myself with the knowledge from the very few wonderful menopause professionals and tried to make it simple and clear. We have much power within ourselves to find the answers to our menopause. I feel very passionate that women need to have access to the many complex combinations to help minimise menopausal symptoms whether it be HRT, exercise, nutrition, or meditation.

Travelling through our middle years can be a great opportunity to reconnect with the essence of who we are, rediscover our purpose - mine is menopause! - and embrace a mindset of growth and possibility. I take pride in how far I have come and use my courage, thoughts, and my flaws to express my passion to break down the menopause barriers. I share my experiences to show one authentic voice and a sympathetic ear, and I shall continue raising awareness. We need more and more women doing so.

This is why it is great to have another voice here on menopause. The menopause taboo has kept women quiet for too long. Change is inevitable for all of us and can often help us grow. Hopefully, reading this book will equip you with a toolkit to naturally transition into a new stage in your life. Although this phase of life can be challenging, with the right support you can take on menopause. This time in life can open up new opportunities and second chances. There is another story for women at this time in life that needs to be told, and Breeda is courageously doing so with *Midlife Women Rock*.

Meg Mathews

Author of *The New Hot: Taking on the Menopause with Attitude and Style*

INTRODUCTION

"If we keep on whispering, we keep shaming.
If we choose to raise our voice, we will conquer."

\- Breeda Bermingham

This book is about power. It's about women's power, about truth, injustice, and courage. It challenges the overwhelmingly negative cultural and societal myths surrounding menopause. Collective cultural shaming of women in menopause must stop. Popular culture's dehumanising depictions of overweight, sweaty, crazy, invisible, menopausal women must stop. We are the generation of women changemakers who can do this. With silence being the real enemy, *Midlife Women Rock* opens the conversation. It aims to dismantle the present-day construction of menopause, letting go of the old belief systems and opening the possibility of a new story for women at the end of their reproductive life. The story to date has disempowered, shamed, and silenced women. The consequences and repercussions of this became clear when women voiced their opinions on menopause on the national airwaves recently here in Ireland for the first time in history.

Women's natural ability to tap into their innate power and listen deeply has been increasingly overwhelmed by science and modern medicine. Quantifiable facts, statistics, and data are important contributors to advancement in many sectors of life, with many included in this book. However, wisdom, inner knowing, intuition, and feminine gifts are not quantifiable. They are developed through life experience. Our experiences make us who we are and can have a profound effect on us. They can help us understand that life can take many twists and turns, leaving us with little or no control. Bombarded constantly with external information, we can forget to listen to our inner wisdom. And yet, by the time women reach their menopause years, they have these gifts in abundance.

This book is a means to uncover an injustice that has limited women's lives and wellbeing, preventing so many from reaching their full, true potential at midlife and beyond. The injustice surrounds the fact that there is no preparation, no education, and truly little publicly accessible support for menopause, resulting in far too many women suffering unnecessarily. Menopause is not an illness and does not have to be constructed or experienced as a negative or fearful experience.

One must question women's silence in this to date. However, mute women shame and menopause have been bedfellows historically, unchallenged to date. I believe once systems and structures are put in place to address this, the menopausal experience can be transformed for most women. We can shift the present narrative. I have witnessed this at the *Midlife Women Rock Cafés* over the past two years. These are free monthly cafés facilitated as a safe space for women to share stories and learn about menopause. With events locally and online, women are joining in from throughout Ireland, along with Scotland and the UK, to support one another. It was not long ago that little education existed on pregnancy and childbirth. Yet, today, information and support are everywhere. Why not menopause?

In 2018, as I perused the menopause literature, something did not sit well with me. I remember asking myself, "Could this be true?" The narratives for women as we reached the end of our reproductive years were so negative and deeply entrenched with the ideas of crisis, loss, degeneration, disease, the best behind us. None of this resonated with me. I have worked with women for years, particularly mothers, and my experience has been one of observing women meet various challenges and overcome them with the right support and understanding. Why is menopause any different? Systematic endemic taboo, silencing, and shaming women is a massive contributor. Confronting a taboo subject is never easy, I knew it was not going to be easy. With *Midlife Women Rock* I am challenging decades and decades of social conditioning and placid acceptance of social norms concerning women who have reached the end of their fertile years.

The social scientist, Brené Brown, and historian, Professor Mary Beard, both refer to shame and stigma in their work. Where shame lurks, it is too often used as a regulating tool, creating conformity, and ensuring adherence to social norms, in this case, women's silence. Women feel ashamed to be menopausal, fearful and in denial, thus we stay quiet. From reviewing the research over the past few years along with conducting my research in 2020 *(Silence, Taboo and Midlife Women)*, Shame, fear, denial, stigma and isolation are narratives that continue to be associated with this life transition. The impact has been to shut down women's voices and deny them agency at this time in their life. When I refer to 'agency', I mean our capacity to act independently, to find our own answers to issues that affect us, and to make our own free choices so as not to follow social or generational norms. No one is denying menopause symptoms can be debilitating. However, by providing education, preparation, and information, the lived experience can be transformed from the overwhelmingly negative. I have witnessed this at the *Midlife Women Rock Cafés*. We must start by removing the silence. A revolution is needed.

Normalising conversations, nationwide awareness, and education campaigns, along with correctly supporting women can lead to a reconstruction and re-characterisation of the menopause story. As women journey through these years, a story filled with new possibilities, opportunities, second chances, and access to deep creative power is a possibility for all. This story sits within the literature, but for too long it has been overshadowed by the crisis, loss, and degenerative rhetoric.

Menopause is a highly significant transition in a woman's life. Trivialised and neglected to date, it occurs as women reach the end of their reproductive years. By 2030, it is estimated the world population of menopausal women will be over 1.2 billion with 47 million entering perimenopause annually. The average age a woman reaches menopause is 51. Every woman transitions through this life phase, unlike pregnancy and childbirth, yet publicly accessible information and understanding remains abysmal. Provision of this will be transformative.

I write from a woman-centric perspective. I am a woman, mother, daughter, wife, sister, and friend. This book provides a general overview on the stages, symptoms, and management pathways available. It investigates how silence and shame became synonymous with menopause. Within these pages, women are encouraged to become the C.E.O.'s of their health, to challenge cultural and intergenerational mindsets around this life stage and in doing so, uncover cultural and societal truths leading to paradigm shifts for women. It has evolved from my own menopause journey along with my life and work experience, having worked with women for decades as a nurse, and most recently as a menopause coach.

I have witnessed remarkable transformation in women once they are informed and understand the physical, psychological, emotional, and spiritual dimensions to this journey. Information and understanding oneself at this phase of life changes everything and gives women access to powerful agency.

Poor emotional and mental health interferes with our ability to actualise our full potential and find meaning, love, and fulfilment in life. Empowerment at midlife comes from validation of life experience (everything that has happened in your life to date has made you who you are) coupled with an inner sense of wisdom.

You will hear women's stories and voices throughout this book. As Elizabeth Lesser says in her book, *Cassandra Speaks*, when women are the protagonists in a story, cultural human stories that have been blindly handed down from generation to generation can be changed. I genuinely believe it is in sharing our stories that we will enable others to realise they are not alone, along with changing the story to date from denigration to possibilities.

Midlife Women Rock is the culmination of three years of researching, my own menopause journey, and the menopause stories of some of the hundreds of women I have had the privilege of encountering on their journeys. There is an academic and working life perspective interwoven throughout this book, but it is written for everyday women, by a woman who had to become a detective to gather all the pieces of the jigsaw puzzle called menopause. It is a story that continues to evolve.

At its heart, *Midlife Women Rock* is a book about empowerment and raising women up. It is only when we question and investigate that we can change the status quo. It assists in the unearthing of an injustice that has culturally and societally inhibited and limited women at the end of their fertile years for decades. It reveals the universal power of intergenerational perceptions, mindsets, and attitudes surrounding the taboo of menopause. Furthermore, this book spotlights the detrimental effect of silence and silencing of women who are menopausal, along with challenging media depictions of menopausal women that continue to disempower and disenfranchise. It explores common questions, such as: *What is menopause? What are the stages? The symptoms? What management pathways are there? Where do women go for support? Where do women go to gain a deeper understanding of self during this transition? How can women make self-care a priority during this time when there are so many other demands and distractions?*

Provocative, insightful, and game-changing, this book is filled with encouragement, hope, possibilities, practical advice, and everyday women's stories. It will help women at all stages to take control of their menopause journey and discover the true gifts and superpowers of this life transition.

This book will embolden and empower you to take on your menopause and manage these years your way. The key with taboo is to constantly spotlight the issue until it is no longer uncomfortable to talk about it. We are the generation of women who can do this.

I am an unapologetic disruptor, on a mission to disrupt the way menopause has been framed for decades, one that has not served women's best interests. We need to break away from the shame and the old story. It has limited us and kept us invisible for far too many years. We need to realise that the system has let down far too many women to date. Keep talking or start talking openly, this is how we break down the power of taboo.

As a firm believer in the power and potential of creating change, I am adamant we can all contribute to the growing midlife women's movement and add to those who are already amplifying their voice for change. Passionate about collaborating with women, I believe in the power of every woman to find the answers she needs to support herself through her menopause years. New opportunities, second chances, access to a deep creative power, courage, and innate leadership potential await as we move through these years.

PART ONE

WE NEED TO TALK ABOUT MENOPAUSE

CHAPTER 1

WHY WE NEED TO TALK ABOUT MENOPAUSE

*"Silence afflicts too many women's lives –
the silence that keeps women from expressing themselves freely,
from being full participants even in the lives of their own families."*

\- Hillary Rodham Clinton

Scanning the room as I walked into the Meg Mathews *Megs Menopause* conference in May 2019, my bold, courageous heart thumped as I entered unknown territory. A conference on menopause organised by women for women. Unheard of globally before this. Here I was in a room full of quietly inquisitive women wanting to learn more about a transition in life every woman moves through. As I sat uncomfortably not knowing what to expect, Meg and Caroline Gaskin warmly welcomed us all and opened the conference by informing us that over 70% of the women in the room had arrived alone. This is the power of taboo, silence, and decades of shame.

Normally women attend events with friends or in groups. Menopause is an exception. Over the years there have been many menopause conferences organised by male and female medics which only discussed the medicalisation of menopause. This was very different. Dr Louise Newson who was medical advisor to the conference commented on this. The integrative and holistic approach of the *Megs Menopause* conference spotlighted menopause from a woman's perspective. It encompassed women's lived experience, women's lives in a kaleidoscope of colourful emotions, and all of the ups and downs. Although emotive at times as we listened to women's stories, a shift in energy as the day progressed led to a determination for more conversations and a belief that open information sharing could impact the present-day construction of menopause. Mathews' vision and superb ability to orchestrate such a conference enabled three hundred of us to sit vulnerably yet comfortably as we talked openly about a taboo subject, stimulating much discussion around women's silence to date.

Women-centered conferences and events can facilitate the production of a more positive and enabling cultural construction of menopause. The camaraderie created in the room left us all realising there is a need to explore this taboo subject and keep talking openly. The emotional, psychological, social, and spiritual lives of menopausal women were touched upon throughout the day, which led to a powerfully informative, uplifting, and energised event that had us dancing on stage with the wonderful Michelle Zelli at the end of the day.

Over the past two years, the United Kingdom (UK) has been leading the way in attempting to ensure menopause becomes normalised in public discourse. Society's reluctance to openly discuss this time in a woman's life has contributed massively to how we navigate this life stage. Today, we have the greatest cohort of women entering and moving through their 50s who are educated, economically independent, and in the workplace than at any other time in history. This generation of women deserves a new story that can only emerge when the conversation is opened up. The old story surrounding stigma and shame has limited and disempowered us for too long.

The *Midlife Women Rock Project* began in 2019 as a 60-day posting on Facebook to share information on menopause. Its introduction provided women with the basic information, the vocabulary around stages, symptoms, and management options. With the project, I aimed to share the information I would have liked to have known. Women have often said to me, "You're a nurse. Surely you must have known all about menopause." And my answer, repeatedly, is, "I really did not have a clue!"

Not alone in this lack of knowledge, I have come to recognise the understanding of menopause is sparse even for nurses, GP's, professors, neuroscientists. It does not matter who you are or where you work. I have discovered very few have this information readily available to them. It's the power of taboo, along with structures and systems which remain in place until challenged. Hot flushes were throwaway comments from my mom and aunts that made me aware that there is truly little spoken about menopause. But when I started researching, I was fuming as I unearthed the hidden information, including thirty-four different symptoms with physical, emotional, and psychological impacts. Perimenopause was a word I had not heard of before 2018. Why was this information not available publicly? It is a massive generational injustice to women, relationships, and families. The cultural and societal silence was deafening the more I researched.

> We need to understand the power and impact of the menopause taboo on women's lives on a macro level. It is a societal, cultural, and almost global issue. The lack of education, no preparation, shame, and stigma has to be tackled by governments.

In her trailblazing book, *Untamed*, Glennon Doyle refers to women generally doing "hard things" in their lives. My own work and life experience tend to concur. She goes on to say that societies often need to "uncover in order to recover". As I observe what is happening in the UK in relation to menopause, the unearthing and uncovering of decades of silence are all too real. A grass-roots movement has emerged. Every day, strong women leaders such as Diane Danzebrink, Jane Lewis, Nicki Williams, Maryon Stewart, Dr Louise Newson, Professor Myra Hunter, and Dr Marilyn Glenville are speaking out and providing much-needed information. This movement has gained traction due to celebrities courageously stepping up to share their own stories, including Meg Mathews, Liz Earle, Lorraine Kelly, Davina McCall, Lisa Snowden, and Carol Vorderman. It is wonderful to witness the collaborative effort of women coming together pro-actively achieving seismic change.

Having information and education, along with support, is hugely validating and stress-reducing. The stereotypical construction and management of menopause to date is a massive hidden barrier to women's progression at midlife.

> Collective silence around menopause has, for too long, limited, and thwarted women's agency as well as adversely impacting women's health. The devaluing of our cultural story sees women's worth in society ascribed to childbearing and rearing with very little written on women's roles post fertility. Who are we now? What is our role in society?

Recent years have seen increased levels of attention to women's health issues in Ireland. In particular, women's health came to the fore during the Repeal the 8th campaign on abortion and the cervical screening check controversy. The hugely inspirational Irish activist, author, and cancer survivor Vicki Phelan continues to advocate to improve women's health experiences and outcomes, suggesting a minister for women's health should be considered. Health policies and services need to reflect the different health needs of different cohorts in society. Menopause is an area that has been neglected to date. Women's advocacy has the power to change this. The open sharing of information between women is pivotal to enable us to understand both ourselves and our menopause at this phase of life. There is no template for the menopause journey. Every woman is unique in how she experiences this transition, which is wonderful when you think about it. And yes, it is a transition, a transformative phase of life, the reversal of puberty as we arrive at the end of our fertile years. In this sense, it is an ending. There is a change, and like any change we encounter in life, it can be frightening or scary if we are not equipped to deal with it. Sadly, most of us are not.

Menopause is universal, unlike pregnancy and childbirth. All women will travel through what I call "Menopause-Land", a natural biological process. Yet, it remains a taboo subject in so many cultures, particularly in the western world. This, I have discovered, contributes to increasing symptomology. A paradox exists. The whispering, stigma, and shame feed the existing story. Having open conversations begins to smash the taboo narrative and will enable us to change this story and provide necessary support if needed. There are what I call gifts and superpowers available to us women as we move through our menopause years. The world needs to hear about these gifts, which include increased courage, confidence, creativity, innate leadership potential, and increased self-awareness. Managing symptoms is key to enabling women to access these opportunities and second chances. Investing in ourselves also helps.

Education and widely accessible information is the first step needed to change the old story.

> Cultural shifts and story challenges occur slowly. The good news is that change is occurring because the truth is, there is no longer any need to feel shame, fear, or denial when we reach the door of perimenopause.

CHAPTER 2

WELCOME TO MENOPAUSE LAND

"Optimism is the faith that leads to achievement.
Nothing can be done without hope and confidence."

- Helen Keller

I arrived at perimenopause unprepared, uneducated, uninformed, and in shock at the massive lack of information. Over the past three years, I have continually asked myself and others, how could this have happened? As mentioned at the outset, I see it as a grave injustice to women and societies. The hidden societal structures and systems which enable the silence, shame, fear, and denial to thrive must be challenged. We cannot solve a problem we cannot see, so opening the conversation is key. Keep talking. This is how we smash taboo!

When, as girls, we reach puberty, our hormonal world kicks off, and for the next thirty-five-plus years we are influenced by these hormones. When we arrive at the door of perimenopause, the reverse happens. Menopause is like puberty in reverse. The hormones which played a huge and necessary role in our reproductive years start to fluctuate and diminish, leading to turbulence for many. Statistics point to 80% of us experiencing some symptoms at this life stage, with 20% adversely affected.

Hormones are particularly important in women's lives at midlife, but there is much more to us. Shifting present-day, predominantly negative mindsets surrounding menopause can be powerfully transformative. Hormone replacement either naturally (supplements or food) or through medically prescribed hormones (HRT) plays an integral role in managing symptoms and in preventative healthcare. However, our mindsets, feelings, emotions, attitudes, opinions, life experiences, and agency all contribute to the navigation of this transition. Terminology and language used about this phase of life is explained in the next section with statistics utilised to highlight the importance of bringing this conversation into the public arena. Let's dig in and understand the language of menopause.

THE LANGUAGE AND STAGES OF MENOPAUSE

Societal structures, silence, taboo, and minimal female-centric research have contributed to women not having readily available appropriate language and vocabulary. As a result, it is only in the past few years that I have become acquainted with most of this language.

What is Menopause?

Menopause is a highly significant natural transition in a woman's life, marking the end of her reproductive life and the start of a new chapter with opportunities and second chances. It's a general umbrella term used to signify this ending of a woman's fertile years. It is not a disease or an illness. It is retrospectively diagnosed. Therefore, we have to look back over the past 12 or 24 months to understand what stage of menopause we are at, which can be tricky and confusing for us.

To clarify, a woman reaches menopause when she has had:

- 12 consecutive months with no period if over 50
- 24 consecutive months if under 50.

The day after the 12 or 24 months a woman is period-free, she is said to be in menopause. And the day after this is when a woman is considered to be post-menopause. She is post-menopause for the remainder of her life. The average age of menopause is considered to be 51; however, in saying that, I have met women ranging in age from 38 to 60 at menopause who have reached that post-menopause day. Every woman is unique.

Culturally and societally, the significance and meaning of this transition has been trivialised to date. The intergenerational wall of silence around this time in life has caused much confusion, ignorance, and unnecessary suffering and must be removed. When I first heard the term perimenopause in a research paper, I was perplexed - why I had never heard anyone use this word before?

What is Perimenopause?

Perimenopause is the phase leading up to the cessation of a woman's period, the mid to late 40s being the average time frame a woman enters this period of her life. Knowledge and understanding continue to evolve here. Our hormones begin to fluctuate daily, surging one day and declining the next as the ovaries' production of hormones declines. It is essential to mention here that once the ovaries no longer produce hormones, the adrenal glands can take over, producing low levels of hormones. The body is very cleverly designed. Furthermore, small amounts of oestrogen continue to be produced in fat cells. This may account for the weight gain many women experience during these years. If adrenal fatigue (adrenal glands no longer working optimally due to prolonged stress) occurs, and women are exhausted entering perimenopause, the adrenal glands are deficient in oestrogen resulting in more severe symptoms. Unfortunately, they are not available to help us out. I have met many women exhausted in perimenopause who have found hormone replacement (natural or prescribed) dramatically reduces symptoms within days of supplementing. Perimenopause can last from between two to eight years, with no two women experiencing the same set of symptoms.

Perimenopause is pivotal to understand as most of the physical and psychological symptoms that arise during this phase are far too often misdiagnosed as something else (too often depression or anxiety disorder). I have met many women moving from medical specialist to specialist with a list of unexplained symptoms to be diagnosed as perimenopausal eventually. The fact that we do not talk openly is a massive factor in misdiagnosis and misunderstanding.

What Is Early Menopause?

Early menopause is the term used to describe menopause occurring before the age of 40. The ovaries do not produce or stop producing eggs. In over 80% of cases, women never really learn why. However, some diseases can be associated with premature menopause, such as Diabetes, Thyroid Disease, Pernicious Anaemia, Lupus, and Rheumatoid Arthritis. It often occurs with little warning and may have a devastating impact on women in their 20s and 30s impacting their fertility as they deal with the physical and psychological symptoms which friends have no idea about. Finding support and someone to talk to is vital. Understanding what is happening to one's body is important. Early menopause remains an under-researched area, with 1% of women under 40 in the UK diagnosed with early menopause. There are, unfortunately, no Irish statistics currently available. *The Daisy Network* provides support education and information for women suspecting or diagnosed with early menopause. Dr Nick Panay and the international menopause society have commissioned several experts to research further premature ovarian insufficiency and failure, which come under the umbrella of early menopause.

What is Post-Menopause?

Post-Menopause is defined as the day after you have reached menopause, which medically is once you have had 12 consecutive months period-free if over 50 and 24 months period-free if under 50. You are then post-menopause for the remainder of your life.

For a majority of women, symptoms start declining here. As life expectancy continues to increase, women can expect to spend more of their lives period-free, possibly up to 40 years. Once symptoms are manged, it makes sense that midlife is a super opportunity to focus on health and health prevention strategies.

Having knowledge and support publicly available is imperative. I love anthropologist and trailblazer Margaret Mead's description of this time as "menopausal zest". Women need to be supported through perimenopause to enjoy this zest.

What is Surgical or Medical Menopause?

Surgical and medical menopause is different from natural menopause. Surgical menopause can be triggered by removing both ovaries, as the ovaries produce oestrogen, progesterone, and testosterone.

Having your uterus or womb removed (a hysterectomy) while retaining your ovaries does not lead to menopause. However, there is some research to suggest a woman may reach menopause earlier than the average age of 51. Once the ovaries are removed in your 20s, 30s, or 40s, hormone replacement is key to ensuring symptoms are minimised and health protected.

Medical menopause involves the medical shutdown of the ovaries. Hormones are no longer produced. Radiation and chemotherapy for cancer treatment can lead to this abrupt menopause. Information, understanding, and support are pivotal to enabling women, their partners, and their families to navigate this time in their lives. Sadly, far too many women report minimal preparation and information available, with many wishing they were forewarned and forearmed before surgery or treatment. Bringing the conversation mainstream will ensure these women are supported.

The Mac Study, www.macstudy.ie, has commenced in the Mater Hospital in Dublin, Ireland. The study is designed to try and improve quality of life for patients experiencing hot flushes or night sweats after a cancer diagnosis and for whom HRT is not generally recommended.

DIAGNOSIS

How Do I Know I Have Reached Menopause?

The first thing to say is that it is a retrospective diagnosis. In other words, you only know you have reached menopause by looking back to a year after you have had your last period if over 50 and two years if under 50.

> For the majority of women experiencing natural menopause (non-surgical or medical), clinical symptoms and bodily changes are the first signs. Irregular or cessation of periods accompanied by hot flushes, night sweats, sleep disturbance, anxiety, or just not feeling like oneself heralds that one has arrived at the great perimenopausal door.

There is no turning back now. Those reading this who have just arrived, or are not yet here, be reassured there is nothing to fear. Reaching out for support, talking to someone, and becoming informed will help demystify this taboo subject. The truth is, knowledge is power, which leads to better management of this life phase.

Blood Test

Before the age of 45, there is merit in having a blood test to check your levels of Luteinizing Hormone (LH) and Follicle Stimulating Hormone (FSH). These are two power hormones produced in the brain which directly impact our ovaries to produce oestrogen, progesterone, and testosterone. These two hormone levels are normally low but increase and remain elevated once oestrogen and progesterone in the circulating bloodstream decline.

After 45, our hormones are fluctuating throughout the day. The general consensus appears to suggest that a one-off blood test is of little use. Once you have reached post-menopause, the levels of FSH and LH will remain permanently high. For women with the Mirena contraceptive coil in situ who may be anxious to know if they have reached menopause, a blood test may help.

SYMPTOMS

Symptoms associated with this life transition are dependent upon many variables. Overall health, lifestyle, stressors, mindsets around aging, along with fluctuation, and then decline in our ovarian hormones. Imbalances in the hormones cortisol and insulin also impact this life stage. No two women present with the same set of symptoms, which can add to the complexity of management. Most symptoms appear in perimenopause and decline once you reach post-menopause. There is no research yet published on why symptoms vary from woman to woman. When I started researching menopause, I heard of only a few symptoms you may also be familiar with - sweats and flushes. However, when I learned that there are 34 possible symptoms associated with perimenopause and menopause, to say I was taken aback is an understatement.

> Why had nobody told me about the 34 varying symptoms? Why had I not read this on a GP surgery information board, in a leaflet, a book, journal, or magazine? Why all the silence? Every woman travels through this, and yet there is a massive scarcity of information.

This list may look daunting, but rest assured everything is covered here to enable women join the dots, particularly in early perimenopause and before any diagnosis occurs. We need to understand our bodies at this stage of life. This is key. You may have some, all, or none of these symptoms. Every woman is different. Keep remembering you are unique. If you would like to receive a copy of these symptoms to your mail, connect with me at breeda@midlifewomenrockproject.com The list is great to have in your office, kitchen, or bedside locker. You can share the link with friends whom you may feel would benefit from this.

Most Common Symptoms

Irregular periods
Hot flushes
Night sweats
Sleep disturbance
Loss of libido

Physical Symptoms

Weight gain
Irregular heartbeat or palpitations
Bladder problems
Hair loss
Tiredness or no energy
Dizziness
Body odour
Bloating
Brittle nails
Allergies
Osteopenia/Osteoporosis

Psychological Changes

Mood swings
Irritability
Anxiety
Poor concentration
Brain fog
Depression
Anger or rage

Other Symptoms

Headaches or migraine
Tinnitus
Breast pain
Joint pain
Burning mouth or tongue
Dental and gum issues
Dry and itchy skin
Muscle spasm
Digestive upsets
Tingling extremities
Electric shock

STATISTICS ON MENOPAUSE AND MIDLIFE WOMEN

The world's present population is over 7.5 billion, and 50% of the population is female. The United States alone has 50 million women over the age of 51 in 2020. The world population of menopausal women is increasing. Over the coming decade, global estimates suggest that over 47 million women will enter different stages annually. In Ireland, there are over 400,000 women presently navigating this journey, along with 13 million in the United Kingdom. 1 in 100, which is 1% of women in the UK experience early menopause before age 40. Menopause is not an "old" woman's issue but a woman's issue.

Women over 50 are the fastest growing cohort in the workplace today. Yet, a recent UK report showed that 900,000 women quit their jobs in 2019 due to menopause-related issues. This transition of a woman's life is an increasing force for economies and societies to take note of. Attending an online workshop organised by Channel 4, I discovered only 10% of organisations and companies in the UK have menopause policies. However, this is increasing from a very low bar. In Ireland, it is less than 1%.

Economic factors, rather than soundbites, influence policy change. A recent Forbes report alluded to the global economic cost of menopause being estimated at around 150 billion dollars annually. It is the first publicly available commentary on the costs of menopause to economies. Unfortunately, cultural, societal, and generational silence, fear, and shame have fed many of these statistics. Something has to change!

The statistics are revelatory as the information, education, and supports available are abysmal for women who need help at this time in life. Seismic societal change is needed.

CHAPTER 3

SARAH'S STORY

My name is Sarah. I am a 49-year-old full-time, stay-at-home mum. I live with my partner and my two daughters. I like writing, reading, and recently started sea swimming which I really enjoy. I worked in healthcare for many years but left work a few years ago exhausted and burned out as my mental health was affected. I have attended three *Midlife Women Rock Cafés*. Prior to attending the cafés, I thought how I would experience menopause would be potluck and random for me. But now I realise I have control, the knowledge, the strategies, and I know how to access help. It seems so much more manageable.

BB: Hi Sarah. I am exploring how women in Ireland understand, experience, and negotiate menopause. Can I ask, what was your understanding and experience of menopause prior to attending the café? Where did you get your information?

Sarah: I suppose I felt I had very little knowledge. I associated it with older women at work. I did not really have any interest in knowing about it. I used to hear the women at work make a joke about opening the windows and having flushes. My own mother never talked about it, my friends never mentioned it, but looking at their age, they must have been going through it.

What's interesting is that I was doing a lot of research on mental health and never came across any mention of menopause and mental health.

BB: What made you decide to attend the café? What were your expectations?

Sarah: My period had become irregular. I had noticed I had become increasingly more irritable and impatient with little things. I was kind of exploring whether it could be the start of menopause but was not sure. I wanted some information. I was wondering, was this my mental health or menopause? Just curious.

BB: Who do, or did you talk to about how you were feeling during this life transition?

Sarah: Apart from my partner, I really did not talk to anybody before I met you at the café and now, I can hardly stop talking (laughing).

BB: How did you feel that first morning walking into the café?

Sarah: I looked forward to getting some information and asking questions. I did not really know what to expect, but it was so relaxed. The women were very welcoming and so open. I felt like here we were, a group of women all in the same position in life chatting and supporting one another. The shared experience was powerful.

BB: How did you feel about the experience of sitting with other women listening and sharing stories on this time in life?

Sarah: Having gone to a couple of the cafés now, it's the information sharing at this point in my life that's making a difference. Look at when you became a new mother; there was loads of information and support. You get all of this information about how things are going to change in your life or may change or whatever. Or even as a parent of your first young child, I remember something would happen, and I would think, "Is there something wrong with my child?", "Is there something wrong with me?" and once you say it to another mother, she might say I did or felt like that too. It's completely normal. The relief is huge.

Going to the cafés reminds me of this sharing. How I am feeling at the cafés and having it validated by another woman sitting beside me is powerful and a huge relief to me. Oh my God, it's not only me! I am not the only person feeling like this. When another woman says I do too, or I feel like that too, it's huge. I am also learning from the tips and ideas shared on managing symptoms. They have been great. There is something empowering about sitting with a group of women, listening, learning, and sharing.

BB: That's a very good analogy Sarah. I can remember that relief talking to other mothers.

Sarah: I know not everyone wants to talk, but that overwhelming feeling of not understanding what's going on can be terrifying. You ask yourself, is there something wrong with me. That's why I really like the information sharing. I now know these are symptoms of menopause. It's a stage; it will pass. It is de-personalising it for me. I feel I am getting braver in talking now after attending the cafés.

BB: De-personalising menopause from you as a person? Is that what you mean?

Sarah: Yes. I now know that women need to understand that the symptoms, all those feelings we have like we feel we are going crazy, are associated with our hormones changing at this time of our lives. It's good to understand this, to make sense of it. It's not me personally. This had reduced some of the stress for me.

The whole café idea is so casual; although it's facilitated, it's non-performative. All of us women are on the menopause journey, eager to learn more. The other women were lovely and so open. It has genuinely given me a much more positive outlook. I see in my own life so many women who do not want to go there. I feel lucky to have found this group of women.

BB: What effect did attendance at the café have on your understanding of A. menopause, B. yourself. Has it helped?

Sarah: It is changing my life. The anger I was experiencing. I didn't understand where it was coming from, but when I heard that this is a symptom of fluctuating hormones in perimenopause and that it does pass, to be kinder to ourselves, it was phenomenal to hear that. It's so scary. I have lost control a few times and ended up screaming at my teenagers. It's lucky that I have a good relationship with them as afterward I talk to them. It's trying to understand myself. It can be frightening. Knowing it's a symptom and it's not me is huge. It de-personalises it, as I said. The overwhelming feeling of not knowing what's going on or being on your own asking, "What is happening to me? Why am I feeling like this?" is frightening. The access to information that is provided at the café reduces our stress levels or a layer of stress. Information and knowledge massively help in reducing stress. Not understanding or not knowing what is going on is adding to anxiety and stress levels.

Another issue that needs to be talked about is the narrative of self-deprecation - making jokes, passing insults around menopause. It helps no one. Some may feel it's humorous but is there no other way apart from mocking us, hearing, "Don't mind her. She's having a moment." It's the [idea that] menopause diminishes who you are as a person. It's condescending.

What I am also learning about myself is the importance of the self-care bit. I do feel a lot of us women lose touch with who we are due to the multitude of responsibilities we carry. We deny a lot of the inner stuff, like intuition, due to doing, doing, all of the time. I am conscious of slowing down now, and it does make a difference.

BB: What have you learned or taken away with you that you could pass on to others, friends, sisters, daughters?

Sarah: It has made me look forward to the next phase of my life. What you are sharing about the effect our mindsets have on so much in life was very big for me. I left that first café feeling confident I could take control of this life transition. I now realise I am not at the mercy of people's often shaming attitudes to it. I have my own. I also liked in the café that it was not about having HRT or not having HRT. Nobody knows what another woman's baseline is. I see it's about providing information to give women the power to make up their own minds, choose what's right for them, know that we can manage and take ownership of this part of our life. I loved that. I was considering going back to university, but my confidence was a bit shaky. Having come to the cafés and being encouraged, I have applied! I am changing direction. I want to work with women to enable them to realise their potential, increase self-esteem. This is another big issue for women in menopause. I am more confident talking. I talk to everyone about menopause now.

BB: Thank you, Sarah. Is there anything else you would like to add?

Sarah: Information and education change everything. Women talking and helping each other is powerful. We need to do more of this. Attending this café has been life-changing. I feel more confident in myself, and in my knowledge base, a huge layer of stress has been removed. Hearing about the positive sides to what menopause brings, I never heard any of that before. Bravery, creativity, the kick-ass attitude, I love that one and can't wait for it (laughing). I feel optimistic about turning 50. There has been a shift in my outlook on life. I am very grateful for this.

Menopause – What Do You Know?

What is menopause?

_____

Can you name the stages of menopause?

_____

What is the average age one reaches menopause?

_____

What are the symptoms of perimenopause?

_____

Can you be in perimenopause at 43?
Yes   No

What is early menopause?

_____

When are you in post-menopause?

_____

What is surgical/medical menopause?

_____

How many women in Ireland are moving through menopause?

_____

What is your menopause story?

_____

PART TWO

RESEARCHING
MENOPAUSE

CHAPTER 4

BECOMING A MENOPAUSE
DETECTIVE

"Understanding the link between women's empowerment and the health and wealth of societies is crucial for all of humankind".

- Melinda Gates

To understand why many of us still whisper or keep our voices down when talking about this universal experience, we need to look at how we arrived here, the framing of the story to date.

During the final year of a psychology degree, I became interested in menopause. I was reviewing the research literature on midlife women, often referred to as an invisible cohort in academia due to little research. Menopause was a part of this story. Many of the research studies did not resonate with me, my life, or my work experience. And so, I returned to university to dig deeper into the research. Many of the findings and voices of women interviewed during my masters research are included in this book. Emerging from the literature and my research is a huge sense of anger and disbelief that menopause has continued to be hidden in societies. Why has no one stood up and shouted, "Stop" to the deficiency in education and support? Why have we remained mute? The lived experiences of an increasingly large number of women are resisting the predominantly negative narrative. Thus, there is a need for change.

When we look back in history, the earth was considered flat for many millennia until one individual decided to investigate, took a risk, and discovered it is actually round. I use this analogy when I look at how menopause is constructed today in a way that limits, disenfranchises, and often dehumanises women (with its comedic depictions of hot, obese, and sweaty women). Somebody needs to shout, "Stop!" I know we can reframe and recharacterise it!

The truth is there is no shame in becoming menopausal. There is no need to be afraid, or in denial, or remain silenced. I started my menopause journey with very little knowledge, but I discovered the truth about this life transition in searching to educate myself. Information, understanding, and medical support for those that need it changes everything (as noted by a Channel 4 documentary in 2021, 10% of women in the UK take HRT). Founding the *Midlife Women Rock Cafés* was an effort to provide support and to validate what I had discovered. I truly believe once women are informed, educated, understand themselves, and are supported, they can thrive through these years. Powerful generational mindset shifts and perceptions around the framing of this life stage need to be challenged for midlife women to live their best lives, which is often discussed at the cafés. Fear and denial of reaching menopause are blocking women from reaching out for help, often leading to crisis. What it is to be menopausal today can be very different from our mother's generation. Still, we must open up the conversation and ensure menopause becomes normalised, just like pregnancy and childbirth. Many of the women I connect with tell me they have never heard a positive word associated with menopause. But there are positives, many of them. They come from the lived experiences of women who have taken on menopause and realised that they could thrive through these years, with the right support. These positives are within the research, but the negative crisis has overshadowed them with rhetoric of loss, degeneration, and disease engendering fear and denial for decades. I have discovered women love hearing about the positives. It changes perspective, and it shifts attitudes. This concurs with the latest neuroscience, neuropsychology, and epigenetics studies on the mind-body connection from Dr Nessa Carey, Professor Ian Robertson, and Dr Bruce Lipton. Our thoughts really do influence our beliefs and cellular metabolism.

I want you to imagine a seesaw. It goes up and down. For decades, the old negative story of menopause with failure, loss, crisis, degeneration, and downhill has been on the upside of the seesaw, sadly limiting, silencing, and stigmatising women. We need a rebalancing. We need the positive story to rise on the seesaw. One about opportunity, second chances, creativity, and courage. A story that becomes a reality once women are supported. Let it be spotlighted. By doing so, we can remove the taboo and open the conversation.

Digging deeper into the research points to the need for urgency around demystifying stories and changing the narrative about menopause. The Central Statistics Office (CSO, 2019) statistics around mental health for women and girls in Ireland are highest in the 45 to 55 age group, with suicide rates for women peaking at 51 across the lifespan. The UK has similar statistics. No research directly points to the correlation between menopause transition and these statistics, in part since this cohort of women is the most under-researched in academia. However, the dots need to be connected. My research discovered the wall of silence as the real enemy, along with a lack of women's voices. We cannot solve a problem we cannot see. Conversations need to open up in safe spaces, including workplaces, and education for doctors and healthcare providers needs to be prioritised for women needing extra help.

CHAPTER 5

FEMININE FOREVER: THE MEDICALISATION OF MENOPAUSE

"For our own success to be real,
it must contribute to the success of others."

\- Eleanor Roosevelt

Narratives of menopause are constructed in medical frameworks and socio-cultural understandings. *Silence, Taboo, and Midlife Women* (2020) explored how women develop their personal understandings, access information, negotiate, and understand different narratives and discourses. It looked at the importance of social support and its impact on outcomes. Having a safe place or space to assist and allow women to develop and express understandings of a taboo subject like menopause is lifechanging.

> Menopause encompasses an arena that is part of a much broader lack of understanding and a shortage of research into midlife women's life experiences. Unlike pregnancy and childbirth, every woman on the planet will experience menopause. Yet, to date, the universal story does not appear to respect its immense significance in a woman's lifespan.

I should point out here until recently, very little pertaining to menopause was written about by women. The pervasive menopause story today emanates from the world of medicine. What was published in mainstream media came from male doctors and professors who wrote for other male doctors looking after a percentage of women who required medical help; very little was heard from women who did not require medical assistance. Their voice has not been recorded (Cleghorn, 2021). The medicalised story was predominantly negative surrounding failure, loss, and madness. In reviewing the trajectory of discourses surrounding menopause dating back to the 1950s, meanings ascribed to menopause have changed over time. They have shifted from a part of a woman's life, a transition like puberty, to a bodily problem that requires special medical attention and treatment. In recent years, some researchers go further. They argue menopause became socially constructed due to medicalisation (Mattern, 2019: Voici, 2018) which removed the conversation from a natural biological process with some negative and transitory consequences that deserved to be supported to a degenerative disease warranting medical intervention. This was a very significant shift as language is powerful. Puberty is not pathologised. Why should the predominant story of menopause be so? Nobody denies there is a percentage of women who need expert medical care during menopause, similar to pregnant women. However, pregnancy is not considered a disease, neither should menopause. Pregnancy and childbirth are difficult for some, but the overarching narrative for the majority is not negative. It is not that long ago that little information existed in public mainstream media around pregnancy. Change has occurred, so why not bring change to menopause? The lived experience of a huge cohort of women is not reflected in the crisis narrative of menopause that still exists.

As medicalisation's sole focus is on the loss of hormones, an increasing number of enlightened doctors and researchers, including feminists, anthropologists, sociologists, and psychologists, argue that the biomedical model has failed to account for menopausal transition in any meaningful way (Mattern, 2019: Gunter, 2021: Steinke, 2019: Northrup, 2021: Greer, 2019: Miller, 2021). As we reach our middle years, many women talk about the importance of reflection, meaning, and contribution, which contribute greatly to life fulfilment. In 2021, the time has come to explore and have open, mainstream conversations around the possibility that there has to be more to menopause than the degenerative or deficiency disease model, which emerged from the medical model. The World Health Organisation's 1981 definition of menopause as an "oestrogen deficiency syndrome" provides credibility for this. It allows for the middle-aged female body to be constructed within the language of deficit, socially and medically deficient, marked by decline, loss of youth, and shame. The lived experience of a large cohort of middle-aged women today is no longer aligned with this denigrating definition saturating the literature – the World Health Organisation needs to revisit its definition in 2021.

In searching for the roots of shame and fear around menopause, enter Dr Robert Wilson and his bestselling book *Feminine Forever*, written in the 1960s. It was marketed as a revolutionary breakthrough for women. A proponent of the deficiency disease model, Wilson saw menopause as the death of womanhood and coined the phrase withered "crippled castrates" when referring to women who reached the end of their fertile years. To Wilson, menopause was a pathological state, a state of illness rather than health. His answer to allay becoming the withered "crippled castrate" was to prescribe large doses of hormones made from horses' urine. He was the first person to equate the ovaries and oestrogen to the pancreas and insulin production in diabetes. We replace the hormone in diabetes, in this case, insulin, so let's do the same for menopausal women. He concluded large doses of equine hormone replacement could eliminate menopause and keep women feminine forever.

As I reviewed the work of Dr Wilson and others at this time who were helping women, many women did benefit from hormone replacement. However this derogative, negative, collective construction and characterisation of women reaching the end of their fertile years became mainstream. Interestingly, nobody appeared to challenge them or, if they did, their voices were not loud enough. In looking at how menopause was framed in the media, which is normally drawn to the negative, Dr Wilson's story made front-page coverage as he travelled throughout the US promoting *Feminine Forever*. His message was, "Women, when you reach menopause, your femininity and sexuality ceases." Your value ceases. If I had been a woman in the '60s or '70s, I would certainly have been silenced. Who wants to admit to being a withered crippled castrate? Denial and fear of menopause became mainstream. The shaming, shunning, and devaluing became pervasive and engrained. Popular culture at the time assisted in the denigration as images of obese, mad, and sweaty women became commonplace. Remember, shame is used as a conforming mechanism in patriarchal structures and systems. It is a tool of control. On reading *Feminine Forever* in the '60s, '70s, and '80s, who would look forward to reaching menopause? Their best years were behind them.

This story continues with an interesting twist in the 1980s. Wilson was discredited after it was revealed the pharmaceutical company who produced the equine HRT paid for his book, the book tours, and helped in promotion. Although he was eventually challenged for associating menopause with the death of womanhood, I would argue the remnants of this framing of menopause persist today, and this continues to contribute to the silence, shame, and stigma narrative. No women's voices emerged in the '60s, '70s, or '80s and his book tours sold out throughout

In the 1990s, Dr Gail Sheedy, in writing *Silent Passage* (1998), attempted to open up the conversation. There is an excellent paragraph in her book in which she said when she appeared on the Oprah Winfrey show, the producer told her that it was easier booking guests who had murdered their spouses than finding women to talk about menopause. Another example of the power of taboo and suppression of women's voices.

The feminist and author Germaine Greer also attempted to spotlight menopause and open conversations in the 1990s with limited success. As a society today, we need to recognise the impact and power of intergenerational mainstream reporting, beliefs, and attitudes. The menopausal woman as a "crippled castrate" has little value in society. This massively contributed to silencing and shaming women. We need to stop shaming. The menopause story is a bigger story than medicalisation. Unfortunately, the medicalisation model, although important, is feeding into the disempowerment narrative.

The women's health initiative studies in the 1980s, and other large-scale studies in the 2000s did nothing to really assist women. Instead, all they did was cause more confusion and fear. Sadly, this confusion often emerges in research studies even today. However, what is beginning to emerge is the increase in predominantly female voices examining pervasive, almost hidden patriarchal structures and systems within women's healthcare and careers that prohibit progression. Caroline Creado Perez's excellently researched book, *Invisible Women* (2019), alludes to this, along with Elinor Cleghorn in *Unwell Women* (2021), Mary Ann Sieghart in *The Authority Gap* (2021), and Paula Fyans in *The Invisible Job* (2021).

In 2021, knowledge truly is power. Challenging old stories enables women to speak out like never before in history. In hearing and listening to women's voices, societal, media and cultural shifts can occur. As with pregnancy, women need to educate themselves. In the same way we prepare for childbirth, we need to become informed and be aware of the physical, emotional, and psychological changes occurring as we move towards midlife. Including menopause in school SPHE programmes as started in the UK in 2020 would be a great global step in the right direction. Open conversations amongst women can be immensely informative and empowering. One never knows how one's own story may benefit another. It is wonderful to see more and more women in early perimenopause courageously reaching out, looking for information and support, taking on their menopause journey.

In 2021, medicalisation and hormone replacement continue to play a role in menopause management. However, it is only one part of a much larger puzzle. Having worked with women for many years and returning to academia to research this time in our lives, I have recognised a much bigger story emerging around this life stage. Today I am back working with women. I see clearly that women are so much more than their hormones. The stories I have been told over the past year provide much credibility for this. For so many, the menopausal transition is elucidated as a unique subjective experience or a rite of passage, which with the correct supports and knowledge, enables women to navigate this life phase successfully, opening new opportunities and optimising health. Assisting all women to access menopausal wisdom with support has to become a priority.

CHAPTER 6

SONIA'S STORY

My name is Sonia. I am a 51-year-old married mother of three. I work as a senior manager with a large organisation. I have recently reduced my hours at work due to fatigue and tiredness, which I now know is associated with perimenopause. I enjoy sea swimming, walking, and socialising with friends.

BB: Hi Sonia. Thank you for taking the time to be interviewed. I am exploring how women in Ireland understand, experience and negotiate menopause. Can I ask, what were your understandings and experiences of menopause prior to attending the café? Where did you get your information?

Sonia: I turned 51 last year. My period had become irregular. Suddenly in December, I could not sleep. Insomnia and hot sweats at night became a problem. They were the two main initial red flag changes. I had very little information on menopause. I knew it had something to do with hot flushes and irritability. I was also acutely aware it was all negative "round downhill", "ageing", and was in denial. I did not want to go there.

BB: Could you say a little more on that?

Sonia: I suppose the perception out there is so negative. We all whisper; there is no open conversation. I never heard anything positive, except I suppose your period stops, and you don't need contraception.

BB: What made you decide to attend the café? What were your expectations?

Sonia: A friend brought me along. She had attended two months ago. She talked about how open the women were in discussing menopause, and it was not all doom and gloom. She found the information shared by you very helpful and enticed me to attend. I didn't know what to expect but felt wonderful leaving the café that morning.

BB: Can I ask, where did you get information about menopause prior to this? Was it from your GP, friends, books? Where did you actually access information?

Sonia: My first stop was the internet, your website, and other social media. There is a certain amount of information online, but I found it confusing, frightening, hard to follow, and often conflicting.

BB: You worked full time, until recently, in senior management. Can I ask, you work in a predominantly female organisation. Would menopause have been spoken about openly?

Sonia: Not openly. But I have worked with colleagues with fans in the room. A few colleagues would have referred to menopause symptoms with a laugh and a joke and a wink. A few mentioned sleep issues. You would look upon them compassionately but move on. I did not really have any information or understand it. No talk about it really; a huge lack of information. It is still very much a taboo subject in the workplace.

BB: You mentioned earlier that ageing is one of the reasons why women don't talk about this more openly it. Are there any other factors that may contribute?

Sonia: I think it's like everything about women's lives. There are sexual connotations, end of childbirth years, what next for us? The whole taboo thing for women in Ireland, in particular, sex, birth, childbirth, periods, and all of that area. This area is still not spoken about openly. I think menopause is just an extension of that taboo, to be honest. I don't know if it will ever change, which is sad really and very wrong for women.

BB: Would you agree, though, when you look at perceptions of pregnancy and childbirth in the world and in Ireland in particular, even in the last 20 to 30 years, there have been massive changes in perceptions when it comes to women and their bodies and body image around pregnancy?

Sonia: Yes, certainly there is far less embarrassment associated with being pregnant. Most women are far prouder of their baby bump today compared to 30 years ago, which is great. The media has helped here also. We have a long way to go before women will be proud to be in menopause, probably a few generations after us.

BB: What do you think about the media and how the media depict menopausal women?

Sonia: Invisible! I would say. I have never seen, never watched anything on Irish television where anyone was talking about hot flushes or menopause. It's just invisible, not spoken about. British TV is a bit more open.

BB: You said you attended a one-day event on menopause. What was that like? How many women were there, and what were they talking about?

Sonia: Wonderful! It was a great, full-day conference in Dublin on everything surrounding menopause, and you could see there was a desperation for information and factual information, all sides of it, the good, the bad, and the ugly. It just brought it out of the shadows, I think. I went there on my own, surrounded by women from different parts of Ireland, mostly attending on their own, looking for information. There is a complete deficit of conversation, and I don't know why this is in 2020.

BB: Very good. Can you tell me amongst your closest friends, would you talk about menopause, or have you in the past?

Sonia: It varies with friends. One or two are very open, but some are very reserved unless you start and say something yourself. Overall a huge reluctance to discuss this transition in our lives. I think the other big issue is the mental health stigma. There is a lot of anxiety and mood changes and mood swings, and that kind of feeds into the mental health stigma that is in Ireland as well, as ageism and feminism. I feel that is another reason why people don't talk about it because it's not great to say I am not feeling ok. It still is not ok for our generation to say it's ok to not be ok, it's ok to talk, and it's ok to say I am not ok. That is the generation behind us. But for our generation, it's not really ok to say I am not ok, and I think that is definitely another issue contributing to the silence.

BB: Thank you, interesting. You said you had symptoms for the past year. What have you found has helped you most?

Sonia: I tried Macca and some other supplements like sage. But they did not help with the severe night sweats. I was exhausted and decided to reduce my work commitments. I visited my GP, and we discussed lifestyle modifications, exercise, and HRT. Once I started taking HRT, the sweats went after two weeks, and I had more time for myself. I also went back to the gym three days a week which is definitely helping my sleep. Women opening up sharing their stories in safe spaces like the café is a great help. We need more of it.

BB: Ok, I think we have covered a lot here. Have you anything to add?

Sonia: The lack of conversation is not helping us women. There is a lot of fear and shame. How can this be overcome? I really do not know. I now know that education and information helps enormously. I want to be able to talk to other people so you don't think you are going crazy yourself. I have no issue about my age, but I would love – it would be great if more people were more open about menopause because at least then you would not feel so isolated. It's a transition that takes a few years. I am learning there are positives which is a fabulous revelation! I think we definitely need to break those barriers down and bring it out in the open. The cafés are a great start.

BB: Thank you.

PART THREE

WOMEN'S VOICES

CHAPTER 7

EMERGING DISCOURSES

"Feel empowered. And if you start to do it,
if you start to feel your voice heard, you will never go back."

\- Mary Robinson

Former President of Ireland

The many discourses emerging illustrate a universal experience. They highlight the true reality of how women are silently navigating this life transition and resisting social norms. The story of menopause is engrossed in shame, pain, and traditionally loss. However, the real loss has been the silencing of women's voices and agency at the end of their fertile years. To date, there has been a huge dearth of women's voices or stories, something which has not served women well. It is in questioning this and ensuring voices are heard that the status quo shifts. The narratives included here are from women living in Ireland, women whom I had the privilege to meet over the past few years since I started this work and opened the first *Midlife Women Rock Café* in Waterford city. These women are pioneers. They are courageous, reaching out for support, wanting to become informed and understand this taboo and time in every woman's life. The majority had never talked openly to anyone before they arrived at the cafés. When I started the *Midlife Women Rock Project and Café*, very little information was publicly available in Ireland. Thankfully, this is starting to change, with more media coverage and grassroots women's voices emerging in this space.

Various recurring themes emerged from the conversations I had with women. These voices highlight the importance of addressing these themes, both nationally and internationally, to ensure all women are supported. Ideas that explore a voracious and often desperate need for information; the pervasive silencing of women's voices; how women negotiate the taboo; beyond the physical symptoms, the emotional and psychological rollercoaster nobody talks about. Many women arrive at perimenopause with no knowledge, no understanding, too often understandably in crisis, and desperate for help. The findings also point out how the power of support in the community, as in the café settings, can be transformative and life-changing, providing information through discussions, story sharing, and handouts. This model is transferable to workplace settings.

Accessing Information And Understanding

The lack of preparation and education to date around this hugely significant life transition needs to be spotlighted and addressed by governments and health departments. Information transforms us as café attendee Helena says, "The access to all this information provided within the café has completely reduced my anxiety. I knew so little. Understanding what is happening to me has given me a whole new perspective. Women do not know what is happening to them, what is going on. Why has this happened? Women talk, but we need to be doing more of it."

As Jill points out, knowing there are solutions and support for how we are feeling is life changing. She says, "I thought I was the only one feeling like this, I felt so alone. Now that I have the knowledge and this group of women, I feel confident to talk and discuss what is happening; I am adamant to bring this out of the closet at work and with my friends."

Not understanding that menopause is a phase of life, a transition that can take a number of years, can lead to much upheaval and discomfort. Louise talks about this when she says, "Being around women in a safe place who can identify with my feelings and fears was such a relief. Justification of all of what was going on for me was big. Knowing I am not going off my rocker is an enormous relief. I feel so much better about myself. I know I can manage this and look forward to the next stage in my life."

This is coupled with a sense of defiance that emerges once women have the knowledge and education. Petra noted how uncomfortable some women are when it comes to menopause. "We owe it to each other as women to start talking," she says. "I can't get my head around it. Every woman goes through it, and yet there is so little information compared with childbirth."

Knowledge gained from attending a safe space like the cafés enabled and assisted many of the women to discuss experiences and understandings with partners, friends, and work colleagues. The information, together with having the open conversations with other women in the café, offered confidence to initiate conversations outside. This links to the growing body of work that is focusing upon the correlation between self-esteem, attitudes, and women's experiences, noting that stigmatisation and silence are consequential.

Meabh was also looking for validation throughout her menopause experience and articulately states, "I do feel many women do not know what is going on with them. It can be frightening. I had been to the GP on two occasions. I knew something was not right but couldn't put my finger on it. I was still getting periods, so menopause never crossed my mind. I was sent for further investigations to another doctor and told nothing was wrong. When one is feeling vulnerable and being dismissed, it has a silencing effect. You question yourself. Is it me? What's wrong with me? Although very nervous about going to the café, it has changed my life."

A dearth of knowledge leads to many myths and misunderstandings, with women often blaming themselves. Rachel lost confidence in her late 40s. "I had a lot of health problems, she says. "I thought I was a hypochondriac returning to the GP over and over." The turning point for Rachel came when she educated herself on perimenopause, attended talks and the café. She challenged and negotiated the silence and taboo. "The realisation that what was happening to me was actually linked to the menopause was like having a light bulb turned on," says Rachel. "When I saw the possible symptoms that you shared at the cafe, it answered so many questions. It's not me. I am not ill. I am not going crazy. I don't have dementia. This is the menopause. It's not me. I can manage this."

THE CONSPIRACY OF SILENCE – FEEDING THE TABOO

Women often try to negotiate the silence and taboo in accessing information. My question in 2021 is, why do we have to continue doing this? Rachel has been seeking out this information for herself and has been attending talks in Leinster over the period of two years. "What I am noticing in the last year particularly," she says, "is the rooms are full." She sees a change coming as women are starting to ask more questions. "They are attending cafés like yours. They are not prepared to put up with debilitating symptoms. They want information. The media has a role to play here. The way menopausal women are portrayed as fat and frumpy or crazy. We are all going to be living longer. There are more opportunities for midlife women emerging. Women need to zone in on the positive side of this time of life. I do see that more focus needs to be put on this, and that might encourage more women to open up if they knew that there is so much more available to us in our middle years."

Women come to the café meet-ups or log on online to talk, listen, become informed, and search for validation on how they are feeling. Maria came to the *Midlife Women Rock Café* to build on her knowledge base about menopause. "Nobody talks about it," she reiterates. "My friends, my family brushed it off when I mentioned it. I came to the café on my own. I attended an event on menopause in Dublin last year on my own. I went to a talk in the library on my own. I did not ask anyone to come with me. I guess because nobody around me was talking. There is a conspiracy of silence. It's a powerful taboo. No one is talking, and I don't really know why."

In contemporary society, it is not uncommon that individuals consistently construct and revise personal stories, and so reconstruct themselves. This is also evident in the findings as Maria recognises when she says, "I am on a journey of discovering more about myself. It started last year when I left my long-term partner. I made the decision and did it. I have no regrets. When I look back, I don't know where I got the courage or power to do it. I could not have seen myself do it five or six years ago. I am putting more energy into me now. I read a lot, and I joined a gym for the first time in my life. Since my long-term relationship ended, I realise I have never been alone as an adult. My energy was always given to others. It's my time now."

We need to understand menopause but also ourselves as women, who we are becoming as we reach midlife post reproduction. This is where understanding the full meaning of menopause transition can help, as Noelle and Marylin outline. Noelle has been taking HRT for four years but has found attending the cafés has done so much more for her. "It's about understanding myself," she says, "and all of what is going on in my body and mind. I know I have not been myself for a few years. Coming here and talking openly with this group of amazing women is a game-changer. I have learned so much about me."

A very emotional Marylin, an articulate, educated woman, openly discussed how she had felt an emptiness, and felt a bit lost for a while. The literature reveals as women transition through menopause, many are led towards a state of limbo, unknowing, unaware of what is happening to them. This limbo, liminal, 'betwixt' state, in-between period, is temporary, yet frightening if not understood.

"I thought I knew what menopause was," says Marylin, "but now realise I really do not have a clue. I am taking HRT for the last few years, and it has helped with sweating and flushes, which were terrible at work, but it's all the emotional stuff. I just didn't feel myself, and nobody could tell me why until I came here. Having listened to the stories from the other women, I can see myself. I was lost for a while but am finding the real me again".

Feeling as though something was missing, she struggled to describe this and pinpoint what was absent. She continues, "There was a hole there, a vacuum, I was searching. I have felt like this for a few years. Along with all the physical signs of perimenopause, this lostness was there. It was hard. I attended a talk by Lorna Byrne, a spiritual healer. She has written a few books on spirituality, but it's not about religion; it's a lot bigger. I follow her all the time on social media now. I really love her messages of hope."

The New York Times bestselling author Dr Christiane Northrup, of the recently updated *The Wisdom of Menopause* (2021), as well as the co-founders of Redschool.net and authors of *Wild Power* (2017), Alexandra Pope and Sjanie Hugo Wurlitzer reveal as women move through this life stage, they have more access to their own power than at any other time in their life. Furthermore, the award-winning psychologist and psychoanalyst Erik Erikson refers to midlife as a time of growth or stagnation. A choice exists. It is not uncommon to see significant changes occurring. Turbulent unfulfilling relationships ending, women applying for promotion, changing career, taking a gap year, travelling, or returning to full-time education. Without support and understanding, the opposite can happen. Women leave the workplace, too often signed off on mental health or stress leave, mismanaged physical symptoms eroding women's confidence. This is why education and support are key and why, in listening to these women's stories, one can see how life-changing understanding and support are.

In the 1990s, Professor Sharon Mcquaide referred to menopause as, "The quintessential biopsychosocial experience, both a crisis and an opportunity." For too long, the focus has been on the crisis. It's time to spotlight the opportunities, and in doing so, we can explode the taboo. In her updated book *The Change* (2018), author and feminist Germaine Greer reiterates these sentiments, highlighting the fact that finding meaning in menopausal transition allows for greater access to our own power, and why women need to become aware of this. The findings indicate that not understanding the process and the meaning of this life transition leads to much upheaval, discomfort, and health issues.

A recent encounter with Maria had her relay how she continues to expand her interests and newfound confidence. In taking on menopause, negotiating the societal silence, reaching out for support, and understanding herself, life is good. Women's voices need to be heard. Interviewing women shows how voices can be heard and how women are making their voices heard, even in small places like the café. Thus, after Rachel notes, "The overwhelming feeling of not realising what is going on or being on my own with these feelings, as not everyone wants to talk, was starting to get me down," she says. "I am so lucky to have found the café. It's a lifeline. The women are so open and supportive. Seeing others feel like this and finding out and understanding I can actively do something about it is powerful."

TRUSTING OURSELVES TO FIND THE ANSWERS

Lydia, who also shared her insights on menopause and the transition, outlines how meditation, slowing down and spending more time outdoors sea swimming is allowing her to understand herself better as she moves through perimenopause. "The anxiety I was experiencing last year when I look back, I can see was associated with my hectic work schedule," she says. "I was going, going all the time. I was the multitasking queen, doing so much for everyone and forgetting me. The anxiety and panic were a wake-up call. My GP offered a script, but I was reluctant to try medication. A friend recommended I try meditation. I started meditating five months ago – 10 minutes every morning – it sets me up and grounds me for the day. I now give myself the permission to take time every other day to get out, go for a sea swim or jog in nature. It has greatly helped reduce my anxiety."

As a social researcher, I argue that menopause is a passage or transformation searching for a new story. I arrived here from women's perspectives, having worked with women for many years and coaching women in recent years. The dominant outdated whispered story to date, shrouded in stigma, fear, and shame is not serving women. The lived experiences of an increasingly large number of women show women are resisting the predominantly negative narrative. Thus, there is a need for change. I believe women, grassroots women, will be the changemakers here. Platforms like the cafés enable this change to occur.

Women are often not only looking for validation for themselves but confirmation of what their mother's menopause may have been like. A discussion which many of the women have considered as part of their own journey is the effect of what they feel was menopause on their mothers at midlife. An emotional attendee outlined this by saying, "The information I have gained from attending the café is not only helping me understand myself but also my mother. When I think back to when she was around 50, I was 18 doing my Leaving Cert. I remember her being so critical, moody, always in bad form (getting very upset). She probably had no idea what was going on. She became very anxious, and has been very anxious since. She never addressed it and probably did not know she could. So much of the suffering is from lack of information and misunderstanding. It is like a negative veil that has hung over us for too long."

DEPERSONALISING MENOPAUSE

This idea of depersonalising the transition from the person ("This is the menopause, not me. It will pass.") is very powerful and was eloquently relayed by Sarah, which we followed in Chapter 3. However, not every woman has this knowledge or awareness. Rachel continued her personal narrative by stating that her perceptions, understandings, and views on menopause have undergone a 360 turn over the past year. "I now see it as a process, not an event," she says. "Women deserve to know this. It certainly can have negative consequences, but education and support help greatly. My children have left home, I am embarking on a new phase of my life, and it feels good."

When women understand what is going on in their bodies and minds, physically and emotionally, it changes everything. Robin emphasises this when she says, "You have this doubt in your head. Am I the only one thinking or feeling the way I am feeling? I was struck by the openness of the women in the café. It felt very safe. I have never been in an environment like this before. It enabled me to share and feel supported."

Other misconceptions that abound include Wendy's understanding that menopause doesn't happen in our 40s. "I thought menopause only started after your periods stopped. I never heard anyone talk about the likelihood of starting in your 40s. It's good to know," she says.

Pam, who left work over three years ago at 47 years of age, very stressed, reiterates the same sentiments as Wendy. She knew something was not right but was getting no answers from the many doctors she had attended. She eventually signed up for a health and wellbeing course, and a woman at the class, who heard her story, mentioned perimenopause. She was shocked but relieved. On researching online, it all made sense to her. "I was so unsure of myself," she says. "I kept doubting myself. I had to leave work. I hit a wall. I was so stressed and did not know why. I thought I was going mad. It was very sad and scary at the time. I felt very alone. I now look back and see it was perimenopause."

What is curious about Pam and many of the women I interviewed is that women know when something is out of balance or just not right for them. The problem appears to be that the answers and support are not easily accessible. Having talked at length to Pam, one could see how she was adamant about finding an answer. She empowered herself by signing up for a course, and she came along to the café because she wanted to learn more. What Pam and many of the other women I interviewed – Sue, Maria, Marylin, Louise, and Lydia – symbolise is access to women's agency. At an intuitive level, they all knew something was out of balance.

My own experience working with women as a midwife and public health nurse reinforces this belief about women's instinctual power. Having access to the right support, information, and understanding empowers women to find answers, treatment pathways, and greater conceptions of self. These women find ways to negotiate the silence and information deficit and actively enable and empower themselves by attending the café.

What is wonderful to witness in 2021 is how menopause is starting to be raised by everyday women in the UK and increasingly so in Ireland. With bloggers, women's conferences (Meg Mathews, Embrace Menopause and Midlife, We are after the Storm), activists like Sally Ann Brady, the *#IrishMenopauseMission*, and Diane Danzibrink, and the *#MakeMenopauseMatter* campaign in the UK. More and more women are coming into this space once populated only by male doctors. Remember what I mentioned earlier in this book about how, when women are the storytellers, the human story changes!

MENTAL HEALTH, IDENTITY, AND MENOPAUSE

Between 2001 and 2018, the mental health rates for girls and women in Ireland were highest in the 45 to 55 year age group with 2016 being an outlier with rates highest amongst adolescent girls. (CSO,2019). Similar statistics for girls and women across the lifespan are reported in the UK. Most women transition through menopause during these years. Helena had her own views on mental health issues and menopause as she navigated her working life. "At work, it's a joke," she says. "If mentioned, it is said in jest, no proper conversations. There is a huge reluctance by friends or work colleagues in conversations. I feel mental health issues at midlife are a big issue. Women don't know who to turn to for help. They think they are going mad, off their heads. Anti-depressants are often prescribed which can help some, but all of this might be contributing to the silence and shame."

Having the courage to reach out for support is pivitol for many, as recognised by Gwen who says she was ruled by fear before attending the cafés. "I had lost a part of who I was and did not understand why," she says. "Tips on self-care and slowing down were good. They helped reduce my stress levels and increase my confidence. I am following up on pastimes and hobbies I loved when I was younger. I have started to go out and meet friends again. The conversations are open, and honest and although it is sad to hear what some women have suffered, we manage to laugh. The café has given me my mojo back."

Menopause certainly is a process that impacts women's identity and understanding of self. Women's identity is structured and restructured in social contexts and in narratives and understandings. Ella found her first serious conversation surrounding menopause at her first café and found she was in the right place. "There was a huge feeling of belonging and connection," she says. "We are all in the same boat. I felt I was taken seriously and felt supported. It has provided a space for me to verbalise all these feelings I was grappling with."

What comes from these stories is the reality that sharing narratives in a group or as part of a community such as the *Midlife Women Rock Cafés* can help in developing, understanding, and constructing identity. Robin found the café to be a refuge for her. "This café is like a sanctuary to me, a safe haven. Women come in every month, sharing and being open with each other. It adds so much to my understanding of me and the menopause. I love the socialisation part of the café. The cup of tea, cake, and the laughs."

The women attending the café articulated very well what the café epitomised for them as Noelle talks about place necessitating agency. She says, "I bring an authentic me. We all have respect for one another. There is nothing superficial about this place. We are all supporting and raising each other up."

Hazel outlined the meaning of the café for her as it gave her confidence along with new friendships. "I go walking with some of the women I have met here," she says. "We have a WhatsApp group. I walked out last month with a spring in my step. I love hearing about the positive side of menopause. It makes such a change from a lot of the doom and gloom I have seen online."

As revealed in many of the above voices, women attending the cafés are creating and constructing new, more powerful narratives within the safe space provided. It is enabling the creation of new meanings for these women. The women are learning about menopause, pro-actively constructing new stories about themselves, and finding the most appropriate ways for them to navigate this life transition. Women feel uplifted. Depersonalising menopause from self provides great solace and reduces anxiety. The findings highlight that in order to share narratives, women need a place separate from home and work. The findings also underline how increasing knowledge leads to greater confidence. As Amy outlines, "We are all equal in this place. This has helped me to open up and keep coming back. I was not judged. It felt safe. With the new knowledge I am learning, I am more relaxed."

Tackling Negative Stereotyping – The Power Of The Positive

When facilitating the cafes, I started to share some of the positive changes that occur as we move through these years. Having never associated menopause with anything but negative consequences, the response from women was remarkable. Petra says she found that the negative illusion society imposes on us as menopausal women needs to change. "Having access to information," she says, "hearing about the positives which nobody ever mentioned to me, educating myself, and understanding what is happening to me is changing everything. The sweats and insomnia can be bad but knowing there is support out there if I need it changes everything for me."

Amy continues by expressing the impact silencing has had on her. "I always had negative thoughts about menopause," she says, "something to be endured. I never thought about opportunities opening up for us midlife women. After a few tough months, attending the café, gaining knowledge, and talking to these other women has given me my confidence back again."

Brigitte outlines how attendance, openness, and access to information can be life changing. She says, "I had these ideas about what it would be like, all negative, kind of all downhill, did not want to go there. I was in total denial. There is something shameful about it. I knew something was happening to me. I have the Mirena coil, so I don't have periods as such. I am thinking about HRT but have not decided yet. From being here with this group of women, the openness, the support, I feel different. It's nothing to be ashamed about. It's only a phase and learning that it can lead to a powerful time in women's lives is affecting my mindset. Nobody mentioned this before. I now see the reality can be so different from what we think menopause is. I tell other women to start talking. This is how we can help each other."

And Lydia, who used Dr Google in researching all things menopause, talks about the power of sharing our stories. "The power of a café like this, I feel is, we are all equal, all on the same journey trying to source information to help ourselves and others. I have friends who would be too nervous to come here, but they would benefit greatly. I love the positive spin and information, especially menopause zest. It gives me hope. Knowing it's not all about deficiencies, doom and gloom might help others to open up and start talking."

This chapter introduced many women's voices that have been absent in the menopause conversation up until now. Voices that are no longer willing to remain silent around this highly significant transition in every woman's life. Let's keep talking.

CHAPTER 8

WOMEN'S HEALTH TASKFORCE

The *Women's Health Taskforce* in Ireland was established in September 2019 to improve women's health outcomes and experiences of healthcare. This is the first women's health task force in Europe. It builds on recent progress in women's health, following a recommendation from the *Scoping Inquiry* into the *Cervical Check Screening Programme* that women's health issues be given more consistent, expert, and committed attention.

To date, the Taskforce has listened to, engaged with, and worked with more than 1,000 individuals and organisations representing women across Ireland. Consultation with and contributions from women is key.

Based on the evidence and informed by women's voices, the Taskforce chose four initial priorities within its action programme:

- Improve gynaecological health
- Improve supports for menopause
- Improve physical activity
- Improve mental health among women and girls

I was invited to attend the stakeholder's forum of the *Women's Health Taskforce* at the Department of Health in February 2020. Credit has to be given to the Department and the then Minister for Health, Simon Harris, for developing this innovative initiative in 2019, the first of its kind in Europe.

The World Health Organisation points to gender as a social determinant of health. Women's health for too long has not been prioritised. The Taskforce seeks to address health issues of importance to women in Ireland. It is a collaboration between the Department, women, professionals, and academics with a remit to develop effective policies and initiatives. It was fantastic to learn that menopause and its management has been chosen as one of its top priority areas to focus upon. More and more conversations are opening up about this life stage, a time that can lead to immense power, opportunity, and positivity for many women once they pro-actively manage symptoms.

From listening to contributions from Orla O'Conner (Chairperson, National Women's Council of Ireland) and Peggy McGee (Director General of the European Institute of Women's Health) along with participating in the interactive focus groups on menopause, it is becoming evident that midlife women in Ireland are finding their voice. We may be the first generation to do so, and who knows where it will lead!

Women's voices need to be heard. The lived experience of women needs to be heard. The ongoing work of the Taskforce is ensuring to include women's voices at decision-making tables.

Safe places like the café reveal how women's voices can be heard and how women are making their voices heard even in small places like the café in Waterford. Thus, highlighting the importance and need for such places throughout Ireland. The narratives emerging at the café have contributed to my contribution to the Taskforce. They expose a massive dearth in preparation, education, information, and understanding of this life transition. A national preventative approach needs to be prioritised.

CHAPTER 9

MEGAN'S STORY

In Ireland one in nine women will develop breast cancer in their lifetime. Two in every three now survive beyond twenty years of the disease. As survival rates continue to increase breast cancer survivors are a growing demographic among menopausal women and deservedly need specialised support. Grief is very natural after a diagnosis; processing acceptance can take time. Reach out for support if you need it.

Megan is a nurse and married mother of two teenage children from Limerick. She tells her story here about navigating breast cancer and menopause during Covid-19.

Megan's Story

"In 2019, aged 52 and feeling healthy, I was gently navigating my way through perimenopause. I was relatively symptom free apart from occasional hot flushes. However, in December I noticed a heaviness and puckering of the skin in my breast. I instinctively knew something was wrong, so I consulted my GP who referred me to the Symptomatic Breast Clinic. Following triple assessment of mammogram, biopsy, and ultrasound, I was diagnosed with node positive breast cancer. I suddenly found myself in an unfamiliar world, scared and unsure of what would happen to me, my husband, and teenage children.

What followed was a series of hospital appointments and tests, each providing more information on the extent of the cancer and the treatment required. The staff were incredibly empathetic, answered any questions, and provided written information on what to expect and how to break the terrible news to our children.

Treatment planned was a mastectomy with node clearance, chemotherapy, radiotherapy, and a 'tablet' for 5 to 10 years. The realisation that I had cancer was overwhelming at times. In tandem with this, the threat of Covid-19 was looming, and I started chemotherapy just as the first wave was gripping the country. Normally, during cancer treatment patients are offered complementary therapies such as reflexology or reiki and the opportunity to have a cup of tea and a chat in the Cancer Information Centre. However, all of these services were suspended. I felt at times that I was navigating my way through it all on my own.

I finished treatment without too many complications. I was familiar with the drug Tamoxifen as a treatment post breast cancer. I was now post-menopausal, so I was prescribed an aromatase inhibitor called Anastrozole for ten years. This drug stops the production of oestrogen. The oncology nurse discussed possible side effects, advised me to keep active, and eat healthily. I really wasn't prepared for the sudden onset of symptoms, particularly joint and muscle pain especially in my feet, hands, knees, and vaginal dryness. For me this was a time I would have benefitted from having a professional to talk to. I felt lost and unsure whether what I was feeling was normal, whether or not to take painkillers and how to manage the vaginal dryness. My own online searches revealed little information and I was unsure what products would be suitable.

It was then I discovered the *Midlife Women Rock Cafés* on zoom. They were a lifesaver, a great social outlet during lockdown. I attended five. Women from many different parts of Ireland attended, some also post breast cancer. Being able to talk about what was happening to me was immensely healing. Breeda and the other women helped me understand the myriad menopause symptoms and what options may be open to me. Surgical and medical menopause needs a lot more attention as it is so very different to natural menopause. I felt less overwhelmed and isolated through the support and safe space the zoom meet-ups provided. The concept of women supporting other women is truly powerful. It provides reassurance that one is not alone with symptoms.

I see a future role for a nurse specialist in the area of menopause post cancer, for women who have finished hospital treatment but need information on how to manage symptoms as they arise throughout the five to ten years of what is still effectively active treatment. Opening the conversation is so important to highlight the need for support."

Megan has since joined the *Marie Keating Survive and Thrive* programme, something she highly recommends for cancer survivors.

What is your menopause story to date? Have you considered writing and reflecting on it? Writing and journaling are terrific tools for insight and healing and can be done anywhere. Why not consider buying a journal specifically to record your thoughts as you move through your menopause years. I call mine my Meno Journal. Keep it beside your bed and add to it regularly.

PART FOUR

BECOMING THE CEO OF YOUR MENOPAUSE

CHAPTER 10

TAKING CONTROL: YOU HAVE THE POWER

"A good leader inspires people to have confidence in the leader.
A great leader inspires people to have confidence in themselves."

- Eleanor Roosevelt

This book celebrates women's innate ability to become the CEO of their menopause journey, to take menopause on. Believing you can do it is halfway to succeeding. When you arrive at the door of perimenopause, having a multistranded SOS toolkit to draw upon is a game-changer. As discussed earlier, at a macro level, the taboo surrounding menopause massively impacts society and women's lives. It remains a barrier to midlife women's social and workplace progression, preventing many from reaching their full potential in their middle years and beyond. A government-led approach focusing on preventative wellbeing and health is needed.

Managing your menopause years to thrive rather than just survive needs a holistic and multistranded approach. Our lifestyle, general health, and stress levels as we arrive in perimenopause will impact our journey. Ensuring we are in good health pre-menopause, just like pre-conceptually, ensures better outcomes and fewer debilitating symptoms. Understanding what is happening to your body, mind, and emotions as you move through these years is a massive stress reducer. As women, we need to understand that we innately have power, and much of this power lies within our bodies. The power comes when we start listening to ourselves. Slowing down, allowing ourselves space and prioritizing self- care all help. This can be difficult for many juggling so many commitments. However, I often use the analogy of the pebble being dropped into the stream-the ripple starts on the inside and radiates outwards. Looking after ourselves ripples in to every aspect of our lives and relationships.

Once women are informed, educated, and supported, I discovered they can proactively choose how these years are navigated. The menopausal bridge can be shaky and rocky, but we can all get over the bridge. The key is finding what will help us to do this. Elinor Cleghorn's *Unwell Women* (2021) tells us that by speaking out and sharing our stories, women can empower one another, challenging shame and stigma against women's bodies, minds, and lives. Furthermore, Professor Mary Beard's award-winning, *Women and Power (*2018) reiterates this with her primary focus again being on women's silence. Mute women and shame are synonymous and are used as a mechanism for control. This is something Beard suggests goes back to Ancient Roman times. This prevailing theme emerges again and again, as referred to in Brené Browne's work in Part One. In reviewing the literature on menopause, I can see much truth in Browne's, Beard's, and Cleghorn's theories. Cleghorn's extensive research suggests bewilderment and confusion often arise when the masculine-dominated medical establishment, influenced by religious, cultural, and political ideas about women's bodies, overpowers women's ability to listen to themselves, particularly with regard to sexuality and reproduction. Handing our power to a masculine-paradigm-run system that has little understanding of the feminine leads to much suffering for women. This, accompanied by the media's double standards in beauty and ageing, means as women age, they are quietly shunted out of the public eye. We are silenced and stigmatised at menopause which is a time when our expertise increases.

The challenge and the answers come from women speaking out. Silence is the enemy. Breaking the silence opens the door to change. More and more everyday educated women need to be encouraged to use their voice to help other women rise. This is presently happening in the UK as the number of women speaking up about menopause increases with the #MakeMenopauseMatter campaign.

Today, if you attend a GP's surgery with menopause symptoms, you will most likely be prescribed an antidepressant or sleeping pill, and depending on the doctor's level of menopause education, HRT. This may well be what many women are looking for and of great assistance. However, keep in mind menopause symptoms are complex, involving interconnected systems in the body. Getting on top of one symptom may bring more attention to another. Having your own set of SOS tools to include lifestyle changes, nutrition, relaxation techniques, supplements, or medication to draw upon will enable you to be in a stronger position to meet new challenges or symptoms when they arrive. Women need time to fully understand both menopause and themselves as they move through these years. Symptoms can change and vary in severity from year to year. Empowering ourselves with information on how we would like to manage symptoms is possible. Start with small changes, set short-term and then medium-term goals, and ensure you reward yourself. Having an accountability buddy, someone to meet for a walk, swim, jog, or to check in with weekly is shown to increase your chances of success by 80%.

Knowledge, awareness, and understanding is the first step. Gathering as much information on menopause as possible helps demystify this phase of a woman's life. An investment now in your health and wellbeing will have long-term health dividends. You have the power to do this. More and more information is starting to become available. The Health Service Executive (HSE) in Ireland is presently updating their website with up-to-date menopause information. The NHS, NICE, and British Menopause Society in the UK also regularly add up-to-date information on their websites.

CHAPTER 11

THE POWER OF KNOWLEDGE: SMASHING TABOO AND FINDING MEANING

"In 'Menopause-Land', knowledge is power.
You better believe it. It's the game-changer."

\- Breeda Bermingham

If you arrive at this book with a multitude of symptoms, be reassured the challenges you now face during perimenopause and menopause are transitory and can be overcome. I encourage you to become determined to take control, and I guarantee your life will change for the better. Removing the silence and normalising the conversation like childbirth or pregnancy can bring change for the better.

We still do not fully understand why women experience menopause in many different ways. Statistics point to 80% of women experiencing some symptoms, with 20% suffering debilitating symptoms.

There are 34 symptoms associated with menopause. Some women may have three or four while others present with many. Keep in mind the severity and duration vary from woman to woman. Some may present with symptoms early in perimenopause even before their periods become irregular, while others may not have a symptom until their period stops. Having knowledge of the possible signs can enable women to understand what is happening. Many women are surprised and often relieved when they first see the list of symptoms associated with menopausal stages. I was one of these women. Perimenopause crept up on me. I was not prepared. It has been wonderful to see many podcasts and expert speakers posting on social media about menopause in the past year. Change is occurring, albeit slowly.

If visiting your GP, nutritionist, dietician, or coach for support at this time, it's a good idea to take the symptom list included in this book with you and tick off your symptoms. This provides a great start to your collaborative conversation.

When interviewing women, denial was one of the narratives often emerging. Women did not want to admit to themselves or accept they had reached menopause. Realistically, when looking at the cultural paradigm around this phase of life, who could blame them? The old cultural, generational story was not something anyone aspired to. However, I have discovered being in denial involves struggling upstream rather than going with the flow downstream.

> Women need to understand that their power comes from understanding the meaning of menopause. Medicalisation has no answers here, so we need to look elsewhere. The meaning of this phase of life beyond fertility and hormones has been socially and culturally neglected particularly in the western world. There is no positive cultural template for the 21st-century menopausal woman. This directly contributes to the invisibility narrative and symptomology.

Cleghorn argues that we need to become aware of the pervasive social reality of masculine power in western culture. The structures and systems in place have let women down and have massively contributed to silencing women who reach menopause (Cleghorn, 2021). In comparison, central American, Mayan, Indian, and Japanese cultures celebrate this time in a woman's life. Opening up an alternative story in Western societies, what feminine power offers (Baker, 2020: Gunter, 2021; Zammit, 2020; Pope, 2017), and what an increasing number of academics (Beck, 2018; Beck, Brewis, Davis, 2020: Brewis, 2020; Krajewski, 2019; Hunter and Smith, 2020) are calling for is a shift from the prioritisation of medicalisation to empowerment and leadership. Thus, enabling women to focus upon the possibilities, opportunities, and second chances this life stage brings. This shift in language from failure, decline, degeneration, and deficiency that populates medicalisation to a language of potentials, second chances, courage, and access to deep creative power, would immensely benefit all women today and in the future. I have witnessed how the shift is a game-changer for many.

CHAPTER 12

THE POWER OF SLEEP: A GAME-CHANGER

World renowned sleep scientist Professor Matthew Scott argues that sleep is more important to our health than our food intake or exercise. Furthermore, every major disease in the developed world - Alzheimer's, cancer, obesity, diabetes - has very strong causal links to deficient sleep. From working with women over the past two years, I have discovered opening up and talking about how sleep disturbances are impacting us helps greatly. Too often, women navigating menopause have no one to talk to, believing that sleep disturbance is something to be endured when we reach midlife. Untrue! So what can we do? Investing in some practical changes, along with reaching out and pro-actively finding what works for each individual, is key to unlocking the door to a good night's sleep as you move through these years. Science has proved taking a 20-minute nap during the day increases productivity. If possible, drop the guilt and indulge in an early afternoon nap if awake during the night. You are worth it, and you have got this.

Disrupted sleep patterns are very common during perimenopause and can exacerbate other symptoms. Brain fog, poor concentration, low energy, fatigue, and comfort eating are all associated with poor sleep. They may not always be associated with reproductive hormonal fluctuations. Women in their 40s and 50s lead very busy lives, juggling families, careers and often caring for elderly parents. High stress levels, leading to elevated stress hormones, adrenaline, and cortisol, hinder our ability to get to sleep. They may cause us to wake often and can lead to anxiety and palpitations, all impacting sleep. When we arrive at the perimenopausal door, this can be an added burden. Like other symptoms, sleep issues are a very individual experience.

Finding your sleep disruptors is the first step in proactively tackling your sleep pattern.
- What is disrupting your sleep?
- Are the sheets wet from sweating?
- Are you worried or anxious?
- Is the bedroom too warm?
- What about excess alcohol?
- Is blue light from electronic devices or a laptop disrupting your sleep?
- Are there issues at work, in relationships, financial worries?

Taking time to focus on your sleep habits in menopause is a worthwhile investment as it impacts your overall health and wellbeing as you age. Focusing on small consistent changes can lead to a better night's sleep.

Let's start with the practical changes that may help.

Look At Your Bedroom

- Declutter your bedroom, bag, and give away old or ill-fitting clothes and shoes. It is amazing how we can feel after a thorough declutter. Marie Condo's research and award-winning books and TV shows on the power of decluttering for modern life have taken the world by storm. The bedroom should be a space you associate with relaxation and sleep. Keep work out of here.

- Room temperature. The best temperature for sleep is 18–20°C. If you suffer from reoccurring night sweats, turn down the heating, leave a window open at night, or use a fan in the bedroom.

- Your bed and nightwear. Night sweats and flushes are amongst the top three most-described annoyances during these years. Consider changing your sheets and nightwear to cotton. Cotton helps absorb sweat and keep you cooler. Changing your duvet to a lower tog may also help. If sweats are profuse, have a glass of water on your bedside locker and a second change of nightwear nearby should you need to change during the night.

- Consider redecorating your bedroom. Paint and wallpaper are relatively inexpensive ways to brighten a room and change the feeling within it. So many women I connect with tell me they have or are in the process of doing this. It is associated with our menopause journey and our ability to tap into internal creative change, which manifests outwardly. You're worth it.

- Technology, TVs, laptops, iPhones, radio, and Wi-Fi can all be detrimental to individuals who cannot sleep. Checking social media before bedtime or when you awaken during the night is not a good idea. Remove or turn off all devices at least two hours before you go to sleep. This helps sleep onset and improves the quality of your sleep. Blue light exposure from electronic devices such as your iPhone or iPad, and laptops delays the release of melatonin, the sleep-inducing hormone.

A Regular Bedtime Routine

Try to develop a consistent bedtime and rising time each day. This helps develop a regular sleep-wake pattern or cycle. What is your wind-down routine in the evening? This is where self-care needs to be prioritised if your lack of sleep is impacting your daily life. Replace Facebook and Netflix time with a bubble-filled lavender bath, listen to relaxing music, read a book, or light a scented candle in your room. Create a wind-down routine and remember it takes time for our sleep rhythms to change, especially if they have been disrupted over a long period.

Exercise

Exercise is great but should be limited to earlier in the day if sleep is an issue. Yoga stretches, mindfulness, and meditation are proven to reduce hot flushes, night sweats, and worry during our menopause years, leading to better sleep. Again, finding what works is key.

Journaling Daily

Another common occurrence during these years disrupting sleep is worry and anxiety. Awakening in the middle of the night with worrying thoughts or feeling like your thoughts are like a hamster on a wheel going around in your head is a regular occurrence. Taking action rather than lying in bed is proven to help you get back to sleep faster. I tell women to get up and make a cup of chamomile tea, have a book to read, or a journal to write in. Lying in bed over-thinking or over-analysing is futile. Keeping a journal for two weeks, writing out your daily routine, including exercise, food intake, alcohol, caffeine intake, work, or family life stressors, and what thoughts are waking you can be revealing. Working with a menopause coach or expert may help you locate, confront or release whatever is impacting your sleep. A great tip from Dr Sabina Brennan and the world of neuroscience involves feeding your brain with uplifting, positive thoughts before bedtime. This feeds the subconscious while you sleep. We have 60,000 thoughts every day, and research points out over 80% of them are negative. Becoming aware of what you are reading, listening to, or believing is the first step in changing your thought patterns. I encourage women to have a book of uplifting poems, affirmations, or stories beside their bed to read before they go to sleep at night. This self-awareness has been a life-changer for many.

My own number-one tip for a restful night's sleep is having an Epsom salts bath with lavender drops added. Epsom salts contain magnesium, which is nature's relaxant. Magnesium also helps with restless legs, another common occurrence during perimenopause. As mentioned above, an increasing number of studies focus on the importance of sleep hygiene and routine. Our busy, modern-day lifestyles appear to contribute to an increase in sleep disruption. Pharmacists and health food stores provide valuable information and advice on over-the-counter sleep remedies. Listening to recommendations from friends on tried and trusted remedies can be helpful. Homeopathy, acupuncture, aromatherapy, reflexology, and Ayurveda can all help. It's about finding what works for you. You are unique. Motivate yourself to start with small actions and you will see change.

Medication Options

- Melatonin is the sleep hormone produced by the pineal gland in the brain. This, along with other hormones, may become disrupted during our menopausal years. Talk to your GP to explore if taking this is an option. Many pharmacies or health food shops may stock natural forms of melatonin.

- Hormone Replacement Therapy (HRT) – oestrogen and progesterone. Many women find HRT the answer to their night sweats and sleep problems. Progesterone is a relaxant. Discuss with your GP if this is the right option for you.

- Finally, cleansing, detoxing, and supporting our liver as we move through our perimenopause is a great investment. The hormones in our bodies are fluctuating daily. The liver breaks down hormones, helping eliminate excess and preventing oestrogen dominance, which may increase sleep disturbances and night sweats. Starting your day with a glass of warm water and lemon helps stimulate your liver. Ilona and Nicki in Part 5 will talk further on detoxing.

Investing some time in establishing a good sleep routine pays huge long-term dividends. In 2019, the National European Healthcare Quality Reporting System (NHQRS) reported that Ireland has the highest rate of chronic benzodiazepine prescribing. The report also found that benzodiazepine prescribing (e.g., Valium, Xanax,) for women over 60 was 40% higher than men. These drugs are most often prescribed for insomnia (lack of sleep) and anxiety.

CHAPTER 13

THE POWER OF COLLABORATION: HOT FLUSHES AND NIGHT SWEATS

Hot flushes and night sweats are typically the most well-known symptoms associated with menopause. Keep in mind symptoms are transitory as our bodies adapt to post-fertility life, with the majority of women who report flushes noticing they diminish after two years.

A hot flush is described as a sense of intense heat rising suddenly in your body to your neck and face, often with the face going red and sweat appearing. Many women tell of the embarrassment of this, particularly in the workplace. Scientists continue to research the actual cause of these vasomotor symptoms that cause fury, agony, and hell for some women. The degree of severity of symptoms ranges across a spectrum. Women I have worked with report flushes varying from a mild breeze once a day to profuse bouts of sweating and flushing four or five times in an hour of every day. They can occur daily, weekly, or monthly, with one woman telling me how she tracked the severity of these hot flushes and how they arrived for a week every three months! Becoming proactive and finding what works for you by using lifestyle changes, alternative therapies, or medication options, or a combination of all will greatly improve your wellbeing at this time.

What Can You Do?

I am a firm believer in the power of women helping other women. The wisdom we all have, when shared, can powerfully help transform the lives of other women. There is no one quick fix. Investigating and finding what works for you is key. There are lots of practical steps which help reduce the severity. Here are some suggestions that help, many gathered from women I have worked with and in the cafés:

- Reach out and ask for help early. Become informed. A holistic, multi-strategy approach works best.

- Adopt a positive mindset and recognise that you will find solutions suitable for your needs. Remind yourself, "I will find what works for me!"

- What are your triggers? Stressful situations, spicy foods, too much alcohol, caffeine, disrupted sleep? Becoming aware of our triggers helps reduce or avoid hot flushes. Organising and planning in advance can also help reduce rushing and becoming flustered.

- Exercise is a pivotal part of management. Embarking on a menopause yoga or Pilates course (online classes are widely available) and meeting women on a similar journey reduces isolation and empowers us as we realise we are not alone. Finding something you really enjoy is key. Exercise increases endorphins improving mood and wellbeing. I meet women who are now exercising for the first time in midlife as beforehand family and work commitments were prioritised.

- Menopause-friendly diets, which include phytoestrogens, soy, lentils, flaxseed oil, nuts, and seeds, can greatly help. Dieticians and nutritionists with a special interest and understanding of the body and gut changes during menopause are an invaluable addition to menopause management.

- Alternative therapies and breathwork, including yoga, mindfulness, acupuncture, reflexology, homeopathy, reiki, and Ayurveda, are successfully used by many to reduce symptoms.

- Professor Myra Hunter, King's College, London, has led clinical trials with increasingly positive outcomes in the reduction of these symptoms using Cognitive Behavioural Therapy (CBT) And talk therapies. These psychology-based therapies aim to challenge and alter negative perceptions, thoughts, and behaviours around menopause and symptoms. This, in turn, can reduce the severity of symptoms. As a taboo subject, it is understandable how negative perceptions are pervasive. Continuing to remove the silence is vital. Your GP may be able to recommend a therapist.

There are an increasing number of supplements available for menopausal women. Finding what may help reduce your symptoms is very individual. In a 2021 published placebo controlled confirmatory clinical trial sage was found to reduce hot flushes and sweats by 50 % after 4 weeks and 64% by 8 weeks. Furthermore, it also impacted psychological symptoms. Magnesium – spray, tablet, or Epsom salts – is used up quickly by the body when under stress which needs to be replaced. Agnus castus, black cohosh, and red clover have been used by women to help reduce flushes and sweats with varying results.

- For women who have "hit the wall" or are in crisis with an array of symptoms, including debilitating flushes and sweats, HRT appears to be the most effective medication currently available. I have met many women who have had good results with HRT and others on it for years still getting vasomotor symptoms. There appears to be no one-size-fits-all approach. You are unique. Non-hormonal meds that help sweats and flushes include clonidine. This is also worth considering if you have high blood pressure as it is not contraindicated. Some anti-depressants prescribed at a low dosage are shown to reduce sweats and flushes. Becoming informed of all the medication options enables you to talk to your GP about the available options that may best suit you.

- The workplace often provides the biggest challenge to many women. Keeping cool is vital as slight increases in body temperature can trigger a flush. Light, loose-fitting, breathable clothes, and layers in winter that can be easily removed are beneficial. Bringing a change of clothes to work is also a good idea. Opening windows, having a fan, and some iced water on your desk are strategies that may help. Planning and organising your week may reduce stress, another trigger for flushes. Having colleagues you can talk to about the symptoms can help while keeping in mind they will decrease in severity and diminish over time. The introduction of workplace policies should be considered by governments as it may help retain expertise. Find what works. There is no need to suffer in silence.

CHAPTER 14

THE POWER OF REMOVING THE SILENCE: ANXIETY AND MOOD CHANGES

Firstly, if you have clinical depression or have been suffering from anxiety for many years, you probably have built up a good relationship with your GP, and they are your first port of call during menopause. However, I meet many women who are experiencing anxiety, panic attacks, and low mood for the first time during perimenopause. It is very common. Many have been to their doctor and been offered a prescription for anti-depressants, anti-anxiety, and sleeping tablet medication with little discussion. They arrive at the *Midlife Women Rock Cafés* or in my coaching sessions, searching for information and often alternatives. Deep down, many of these women know they are out of balance. Something is just not right, but they cannot verbalise why. Many are in perimenopause with the rollercoaster of fluctuating hormones contributing to their mood changes. Denial is common, particularly in women in their early to mid-40s. Others have left work, taken extended leave due to social anxiety, or are self-medicating with alcohol. Many also know they are not depressed in the clinical sense. They come with questions, and with what some call having "hit the wall," in other words "in crisis", and find having a safe space to talk really helps.

I have discovered from my research that anxiety is contributed to hugely by the silence, shame, fear, and denial that has pervaded the menopause story for decades. There is no education, little information, no mandatory medical training for GPs, and no understanding of what is happening to our bodies and minds as we reach perimenopause. Feedback from women meeting up at the cafés shows talking and laughing with other women about menopausal symptoms can be very helpful, reassuring them that they are not alone. In exchanging coping strategies, along with sympathy and empathy, women support and encourage each other to face the world.

As one attendee said, "We know we are in good company and that most symptoms are transitory. Knowing this is a great relief." Women at this time are more susceptible to anxiety disorders and depression due to:

- Fluctuating hormones – oestrogen, progesterone, oxytocin, cortisol, insulin, testosterone, melatonin, or thyroid.

- Stressful life events or multi-tasking for years neglecting the self.

- Other symptoms such as poor sleep, hot flushes, night sweats.

- Lifestyle changes, empty nest, marriage breakdown, or a job loss.

- Attacks triggered by coffee and alcohol.

- The negative paradigm of the "life is over" narrative!

What Can You Do?

Educate Yourself and Reach Out

Women tell me over and over, "If only I knew this was perimenopause. If only I knew what to expect, I would be prepared, I would understand, I would have reached out for help earlier." Talk to your GP, attend a menopause talk, or a café (online or in-person) on menopause.

Avoid Or Reduce Triggers

Take time to find out what may be triggering panic attacks. Are there any recent changes affecting you? Talk to your GP to rule out anything other than perimenopause as a cause.

Don't Dismiss HRT

For women who have "hit the wall," who are exhausted, who have been multitasking, meeting the needs of everyone else at home and at work, HRT is a great start to get on top of symptoms. Looking out for stressors, being kinder, and investing in yourself all help reduce anxiety.

Self-Care, Space, and Slowing Down

The three secrets I share with all are self-care, space, and slowing down. Having spent years looking after everyone else's needs, radical self-care without the guilt needs to happen during these years. It is imperative to understand how you feel because the truth is your health impacts all of those around you – your partner, family, and work colleagues. Working with a menopause coach can help to reprioritise you and your needs at this time of life. Consciously slowing down and giving yourself extra space can both reduce cortisol levels and relax the sympathetic nervous system, thus reducing anxiety. Everyone benefits but most importantly you. The women I work with want to understand what is happening and why. A lack of available information leads to lots of questions that I love to hear. The relief in knowing they can take control of these symptoms is transformative. Many women have no one to listen to them or validate what is going on for them at this stage of life. This is where investment in the self is vital.

Relaxation

Many studies point to incorporating relaxation techniques and strategies to reduce stress levels, thereby reducing mood change and anxiety. Have you considered a daily walk in nature, or by the sea, starting with ten minutes before or after work? It takes 28 days to actively create a habit. Find a buddy or go alone. Walking or fitness apps can be a good motivator. Believe me, once you get started, you will want to increase the amount of time out there. Reward yourself at the end of each week. I started to set my alarm clock for 6:45am three years ago when perimenopausal and I started walking our dog before work for 15 minutes initially. Now, I do 40 minutes every morning. It is so energising and sets me up for the day. Try Thai Chi, yoga, mindfulness, or a meditation class. Many women I have worked with who practise yoga also have a great understanding of the chakra system. It is the body's energy system. It is great to understand this if fatigue or low energy is one of your symptoms. It is never too late to start or try something new. You have nothing to lose. Find what interests you. Be curious.

The Power of The Sea and Forest Bathing

There is increasing scientific evidence on the benefits of sea swimming, surfing, or walking by the sea, to our mental health. The number of women incorporating or beginning to swim in the sea has increased steadily over the last few years. Emerging research also points to the immense health benefits of walking mindfully in nature, spending more time outdoors in parks or forests. Busy lifestyles, and so much time spent online, requires us to become aware of counteracting stress and finding solutions that restore and maintain balance in our lives. If symptoms are severe, slowing down your life helps enormously.

Vitamin D

Vitamin D (D3 Spray) or liquid format greatly benefits low mood and should be taken over winter. Get your blood Vitamin D levels checked during your next GP visit. Sun exposure provides us with Vitamin D naturally.

As outlined in the last three chapters, you can see how menopause symptoms are interconnected, impacting different systems in the body; thus, there is no single overall magic potion or pill that will solve everything. Every woman is unique. Start with small lifestyle changes. You are worth it.

SOS Toolkit:
Wellness Enhancers

Be kind to yourself

Start with small changes

Believe in yourself

Aim for seven to eight hours sleep

Have a well-balanced, nutrient-rich diet

30 minutes cardio exercise three times weekly

Movement is your pill of choice at midlife

Leg squats, lunges, and push ups are great for muscles

An accountability buddy increases your chances of success by 80%

Stress management

Watch alcohol and caffeine intake

Reduce or cut out smoking

Laugh, and then laugh some more

CHAPTER 15

THE POWER OF ANGER: "KILLER WHALES AND KILLER WOMEN"

I have to agree with much of the literature that talks about how uncomfortable societies and cultures are around the subject of women's anger. For centuries, women have been taught that their anger is unfeminine, inappropriate, and shameful.

The predominant narrative tells girls and women that anger is not ladylike, it's irritating, it's defeminising. I was one of those. Raising our voices or articulating our opinions was certainly not mainstream during my school days. In the sixteenth and seventeenth centuries, women who raised their voices to challenge injustices were often associated with witchcraft and burned at the stake. Anger and women today are widely associated with madness. Just look at some of the stereotypical media depictions of menopausal women - crazy, mad, off her head. Social norms continue to dictate how women should express anger which is usually to suppress it at any cost. This leads to widespread self-silencing and health consequences.

Laura Bates in *Everyday Sexism* encourages women to become aware of double standards. Angry women are seen as hysterical, overbearing, or out-of-control, even mad, whereas angry men are often portrayed as assertive and confident leaders. She believes there is potential untapped power in acknowledging and harnessing women's rightful anger. We often have every reason to be angry, and it can be channelled very positively into advocacy for ourselves, in the workplace, or for political and social action.

Controlling anger at any cost leads to unawareness of actually having access to this profound emotion. There abounds in psychiatry a theory that anger turned inwards leads to depression. It is interesting that, in general, women have higher incidents of mental health issues than men, although men have a higher rate of suicide. Contemplating women's anger never crossed my radar until I reached perimenopause. The discourse surrounded the fact that many women arrive at midlife with decades of unexpressed or even unacknowledged anger. As a result of being culturally conditioned to repress or suppress it, a shock factor is associated with its emergence at perimenopause. A deep awareness of this anger emerged and sat with me for over nine months during my perimenopause. I would have found this very frightening if I had not become somewhat of a menopause detective, trawling studies and searching for information. Instead, I was able to sit with the awareness, acknowledge it, believing that it would pass and that it was revealing something to me. Looking back now, two years on, I can see that this anger is certainly linked to our innate power. It's as if a veil is lifted, and we are looking upon issues around us with a new pair of glasses. Our brain, adapting to the diminishing oestrogen and oxytocin, also known as the nurturing hormone, facilitates this. The anger is revelatory and needs to be acknowledged. It does not need to be medicated, suppressed or denied. The science of anger reveals that doing so leads to insomnia, anxiety, and depression. It has highlighted for me the massive injustice around women's voices, agency, and menopause.

The Swiss psychiatrist Carl Jung's theories include the belief that the constant anger and frustration that emerges and remains is like an amber light flashing trying to get one's attention. Something may need to change in one's life. Become aware of anger and irritability if it is an issue for you.

An interesting academic paper by Sabine Krajewski titled "Killer Whales and Killer Women", refers to the wall of silence that remains around menopause. It contributes to disempowering menopausal women. The author refers to the story as becoming a highly pathologised process, orbiting ageing, fears of temporary madness, and social attitudes about older women's sexuality. There is a call out to challenge the social construction of menopause to date. As menopause research evolves, in looking at female killer whales who experience menopause and become the matriarchs of their pods, Krajewski (2019) and Steinke (2019) hypothesise that it is in opening up public conversations that enables widespread access to information and support. This can transform the way women experience "the change" and shift the focus from medicalisation to empowerment. This shift could dramatically impact the mindset of women approaching menopause, allowing them to see it as a positive rather than a negative time in their life.

Recently a friend, on hearing I was writing about anger in midlife women, recommended Soraya Chemaly's book *Rage Becomes Her*. This book calls on 21st-century women to embrace their anger and harness it as a tool for long-term personal and societal change. Chemaly sees anger as one of the most important and influential emotions in human life. Fully understood, it can drive and motivate women to action. Interestingly I have met many post-menopausal women who talk about this newly accessed anger and how they are using it as a catalyst for positive change and growth.

The takeaway from anger research is women should acknowledge it. "I am angry, irritated, and it's OK. I am not mad or crazy!" Understand angry feelings can be part of the menopause experience and nothing to be ashamed of or denied. Having someone to talk to about it is life asserting. One's anger can be utilised in a positive way. It is what has motivated me to do the work I am doing today. A safe community space like the *Midlife Women Rock Cafés* allows women to verbalise their anger, knowing they are validated and supported.

CHAPTER 16

THE POWER OF MOVEMENT: "THE GREATEST SHOWMAN"

Menopausal transition and increased movement should be mandatory. It is the number one healthcare preventative tool that is free and without side effects. The advantage of moving our bodies impacts our mental, physical, and psychological health. Weight gain is an issue for a significant percentage of women. Our metabolism starts to slow down; thus, we need to increase our movement and reduce our calorie intake. If drug companies could develop a pill that provides the benefits that human beings derive from exercise, it would be a global bestseller. A study recently published from the University of New South Wales, Australia, found that menopausal women participating in interval training three times a week for two months showed a marked decrease in negative symptoms. Twenty minutes of sprints on an exercise bike, three times a week, was found to reverse some of the debilitating effects of menopause. Muscle mass was increased, while body mass index (weight) decreased. Increasing muscle mass in our middle years is hugely advantageous to our long-term health. It improves movement, metabolism, and prevents disease. When our body has lean muscle mass, it burns calories and promotes fat loss even during rest. This increases your basal metabolic rate (BMR), which assists in weight loss.

As I moved through perimenopause, I became interested in the science behind the power of movement and how it impacts our mood and reduces cortisol, our stress hormone. I had gained a lot of weight in perimenopause. I will let you into one of my secrets to successfully move through those early perimenopausal symptoms. I discovered dance. I don't mean ballet, tap dancing, or hip hop. I mean literally dancing about the kitchen for five to ten minutes listening to my favourite music. As we head into our middle years, we need to keep in touch with that fun side of us that loves to dance or sing as if no one is watching.

"The Greatest Showman" soundtrack became one of my best friends. I started to dance around the kitchen most evenings, something I felt so foolish about doing initially, but I discovered it works! Many of the women who attend the monthly cafés have also reported seeing the difference this can make. Finding music you love, turning on a track, and bopping about the house, shifts the energy in our bodies and makes us laugh. It also helps us to get back in touch with a part of ourselves we have forgotten by midlife. Give it a go, particularly in the winter months if you cannot get outside as easily. I still dance regularly in the kitchen; my family think I am off my rocker at times! But our dog loves it. Try it and watch what happens. It's also great for our heart and brain health.

As menopause progresses, small changes, like incorporating dance or a daily walk, become habits. Once we start feeling the benefits of the positive endorphin release, many of us then have the confidence to challenge ourselves to try another exercise. There are so many options: swimming, cycling, badminton, tennis. I love hearing from women who are returning to an activity they enjoyed in their younger years - buying a bicycle, taking out a racket, camogie, or a hockey stick from the attic. Preventing osteoporosis is pivotal to keep in mind as we move through menopause. I love a game of tennis, two or three times a week. It is social and has health benefits. There are immense wellbeing and health benefits to incorporating movement into your life at midlife and sustaining it. It is never too late to start.

Exercise and movement also impact pelvic floor health, an area of women's health and wellbeing that also needs to be spotlighted. The fitter you are, the less likely you will have pelvic floor complaints. We would all benefit if we talked to one another more openly about incontinence and sexual health issues. Pelvic floor problems can occur at any age, but as we move through menopause, bladder and bowel problems may increase due to diminishing levels of oestrogen. Vaginal and bladder issues such as dryness, discomfort, incontinence, and urinary infections can affect approximately 35 to 40% of women, and directly affect intimacy. There is much one can do. Reaching out and seeking help from your GP or pelvic health physio is imperative as you may well have another 35 or 40 years of living ahead. In Part Five, Lorraine shares her down below physio tips, while menopause movement expert, Sam Palmer, will discuss the many benefits movement brings along with using movement as medicine during our menopause years.

CHAPTER 17

THE POWER OF UNDERSTANDING: THE FOUR DIMENSIONS OF MENOPAUSE

"Faith is a place of mystery, where we find the courage to believe in what we cannot see and the strength to let go of our fear of uncertainty."

- Brené Browne

The joy of returning to education at midlife is that most of us are choosing to study something we have really given a lot of thought to. Having worked with women as a midwife and public health nurse, I understand why I am here in Menopause-Land. Digging into the research literature on menopause from numerous disciplines and perspectives, it became evident that there are four clear dimensions to our menopause journey, four large puzzle pieces including physical, psychological, emotional, and spiritual. I now believe we need to understand all four to amplify the positives of the menopausal journey. In collectively understanding and consciously managing the menopause experience, I believe we can completely reframe the menopause story. We can move from a narrative of fear, silence, shame, and taboo, to a more open, positive, enabling, and empowering story serving the best interests of women during this time in their lives.

The conventional medicalisation model points to menopause primarily as a physical process, a depletion of hormones marking the end of a woman's reproductive years. Although important, it neglects the mental, emotional, and spiritual aspects. An increasing number of researchers, including many medical doctors (Dr Jen Gunter, Dr Sara Gottfried, Dr Betsy Greenleaf, amongst others), are challenging the trivialising perspective of menopause. It is not just a hormonal deficiency or a disease. Accounts such as this contribute hugely to the disempowering narratives surrounding women at this stage of life. Human beings are complex. We cannot entirely separate one part of us from the other. Each part - physical, emotional, mental, and spiritual - impacts the other whether good or bad. The meaning of menopause encapsulates the four dimensions. The medicalisation model, although important, is not serving women's best interests in only alluding to hormones.

Having become an investigator, examining the literature from a woman-centric lens, I discovered that women's menopause journey varies greatly. It is reportedly seen as a time of turbulence and great change for many, with others feeling very little as they move through these years. The changes are not only to the body but to the brain, our mindset, our emotions, and our spirit. It's a journey that allows us to come into our own as women and tap into a deep well of creative power waiting to be accessed.

I became interested in the spiritual literature around this time in life, which focuses on meaning and purpose. A growing number of studies show that spirituality becomes increasingly important to women in midlife. We need to look after our bodies and our minds. Research suggests that we also need to connect, tap in, or explore our spiritual side, as this can positively contribute to women becoming more empowered. It appears that in becoming enlightened, we become empowered.

Tapping into our spiritual side involves a belief in a force greater than ourselves, God, the divine, Allah, the universe, angels, regardless of religious persuasion. Professor Lisa Miller, Columbia University, has published extensively on the neuroscience of spirituality and the quantifiable effects of spirituality on health resilience, thriving, and joy in life. The British sociologist Grace Davie's extensive body of research on *Belief Without Belonging* refers to the stark demise of institutional religion throughout Europe. However, a belief system does continue. Her research shows an increase in faith unrelated to religious practice. In addition, there are over 300 peer-reviewed studies on the healing power of prayer. Whatever one believes, providing nourishment for our spirit and soul through prayer, meditation, yoga, mindfulness, and retreats, appears to benefit us as we travel through midlife. As we become more spiritually aware, we become more fulfilled, more compassionate towards ourselves and others. Furthermore, Miller's (2021) research shows that spiritual exploration enables women to tap into higher potentials and self-actualise.

My research pointed to the power of preparation, education, and attitude in enabling women to manage this life stage pro-actively. Evidence suggests that choosing our perspective on entering perimenopause enables women to become confident in choosing management options. The problem presently in Ireland and in many countries is the cultural and societal silence. A huge thanks must go to the RTÉ Radio One show *Liveline* and its presenter, Joe Duffy, for allowing menopause airtime on the national airwaves for eight days in May 2021. The voices of Irish women relaying their menopause experiences created a forum for nationwide conversation about this time in women's lives. Opening the conversation is the first step in dismembering a taboo. Sharing our stories can be a powerful incentive for change. You may never know the difference it can make to another woman.

CHAPTER 18

THE POWER OF GRATITUDE AND FORGIVENESS: DOORS TO HEALING

"To forgive is to set a prisoner free and discover that the prisoner was you."

- L Smedes

Adopting an attitude of gratitude or thankfulness in your daily life is shown to increase important neurochemicals in the brain and body. When our thinking shifts from negative to positive thought, a surge of feel-good chemicals such as dopamine, serotonin, and oxytocin occurs. These chemicals contribute to the feelings of closeness, connection, and happiness. Our brains are amazing. Over the past ten years, exciting developments within the world of neuroscience and neuropsychology have learned more about brain function compared to the previous one hundred years. Dr Michael Merzenich's work on neuroplasticity has proven the 55-year-old brain can be as sharp as the 25-year-old.

These revelations help debunk the myths surrounding cognitive health in midlife. When women realise their brain can continue to perform optimally, this massively impacts their belief system and encourages a growth mindset. The inspirational international speaker Simon Sinek often refers to the fact that we cannot hold a positive and negative thought at the same time, so we can choose. No one can be grateful and unhappy at the same time. Danelle Delgado's bestseller *I Choose Joy* is a fabulous uplifting read on the power of choosing our thoughts with gratitude high on the list.

In 2018, The Greater Good Science Centre published a white paper called "'The Science of Gratitude," which outlined the following benefits of incorporating a gratitude practice:

- Increased happiness and positive mood
- More satisfaction with life
- Less likely to experience burnout
- Better physical health
- Better sleep
- Less fatigue
- Greater resiliency
- Development of patience, humility, and wisdom

The study showed that one could start to introduce an attitude of gratitude at any age. Many individuals take for granted that for which we only become grateful for once it is taken, for example, great health, a home, or a relationship. Women I have worked with who have started to embrace gratitude into their daily lives report an increased calmness and peace, along with an increased ability to cope with adversity and stress.

Over the past few years, I have learned and continue to learn much about the menopause journey and myself. Forgiveness was another interesting subject in the research literature, one that is not talked about enough. It is another tool to add to our SOS tool kit at midlife. Forgiveness is hugely powerful, along with being enormously challenging for many. When I refer to forgiveness, it is two-dimensional - forgiveness of oneself and forgiving others. I was unaware of the personal effects that holding a long-term grudge or bitterness towards someone can have. Scientific and medical research points to there being a multitude of benefits to embracing forgiveness. An act of forgiveness can reap huge rewards for your health.

It can result in:

- Healthier relationships
- Lower blood pressure
- Reduced anxiety and low mood
- Improved heart health
- Increased self-esteem
- Better sleep

During our midlife years reflection often occurs, which is relatively normal. Past regrets or missed opportunities come to the surface to be re-examined. Acknowledging these is important. Investing in some counselling or coaching sessions may help to continue moving forward rather than becoming cynical and stuck in resentment.

Nursing has traditionally been associated with healing, helping restore health, and find balance. Having worked in hospital and community settings I have witnessed the power of allowing oneself take time to heal. Opportunities for healing arise as we move through the menopause years with many women embracing these, leading to increased wellbeing.

CHAPTER 19

THE POWER OF LAUGHTER: NATURE'S NATURAL STRESSBUSTER

*"There is nothing in the world so irresistibly contagious
as laughter and good humour."*
- Charles Dickens

ave you ever been in a situation that was difficult or tense only to suddenly burst out laughing? Or notice how good you feel after watching a really funny movie? I am with Charles Dickens – nothing beats a good fit of giggles. There is much evidence and great truth in the power of laughter and humour as medicine. Studies show that as children, we laugh hundreds of times each day, but we have become a lot more serious by the time we reach midlife. Sharing the benefits of laughter and joy with the many women I work with often leads many to comment on their lack of awareness of the importance of enjoying life and having a laugh during menopause. We need to increase opportunities for fun during these years. Once aware, there is so much we can do daily to increase fun, humour, and laughs in our lives. Let's look at the benefits:

- Laughter is scientifically shown to strengthen your immune system and reduce stress levels.

- It boosts mood and often helps us connect with others.

- The parasympathetic nervous system is activated when we laugh, helping us relax.

- Laughter diminishes pain as it switches on healthy physical and emotional responses in the body.

- A good laugh can rebalance both body and mind, lifting mood and reducing anxiety.

- Humour lightens your burdens, if only momentarily. It inspires hope and keeps you grounded, focused, and alert. It also helps you release anger and forgive sooner.

Bringing laughter into your life is wonderful. Add it to your SOS toolkit and draw upon it to overcome problems, enhance your relationships, and improve your mental and physical health. Start with small, aware steps – watch a comedy or catch up with a good friend.

Neuroscience indicates that we can actually trick our brain and move, change, or shift serotonin levels by watching funny memes, a hilarious home video, or watch a puppy or kitten playing. Make it a ritual five minutes a day. Best of all, it is free. I remember the British Oscar-winning actress Judi Dench being interviewed a few years back. She was asked for her number one tip for growing older gracefully. "Laugh. We all need more laughter," was her response. Life is just too short not to! I have to mention two marvellous mothers - Sue Collins and Sinead Culbert, from *Dirt bird Productions,* who are Irish comedy writers and performers. Their regular videos on social media have enabled thousands of us to escape reality in tears of laughter. Laughter yoga is also gaining traction due to its mental health benefits. *Laughter Lab* was set up in 2020 in the UK. It is a new and different approach to boosting wellbeing, managing stress, preventing burnout, and reducing workplace bullying.

CHAPTER 20

THE POWER TO CHOOSE: HRT OR NOT

As a student nurse, I learned that different organs and glands secrete over fifty hormones in the body. Hormone Replacement Therapy (HRT) refers to replacing the reproductive hormones oestrogen, progesterone, and often testosterone to treat debilitating menopausal symptoms. Eating a diet of phytoestrogen-rich food or taking a natural phytoestrogen supplement like red clover can greatly help some women's symptoms. However, it has to be remembered we are all unique. No two women will present with the exact same set of symptoms. Many women may have tried alternatives and lifestyle changes to help with debilitating symptoms, but they persist.

Women need to become aware that they do not have to put up with severe symptoms which dramatically impact their quality of life. We deserve to thrive, not just survive our menopause years. This is when HRT can be most beneficial. Although not without risk, it is the most effective medical treatment for symptoms. Making an informed choice, weighing up the pros and cons can be empowering. Women often trial HRT for three to six months and decide for themselves whether to continue or not. Many begin treatment, and once symptoms are controlled over a few years, they slowly wean themselves off. Others start and stay on it for life. The bottom line is about informed choice and personal preference. Some women will choose HRT others won't, and that's OK. It should not be a "them versus us" mentality. This is an old argument that has never helped women. A collaborative approach ensuring women have an SOS toolkit filled with different management options is a win-win for all women.

Many forms of body identical HRT are available today and are safer with fewer side effects than the synthetic or compounded HRT of old. HRT has been followed with controversy for decades, as discussed in *Feminine Forever* in Part Two. Many studies in the 1990s and 2000s created fear and confusion, again not benefitting women. Opening the conversation about this management option will help demystify many myths. Talking to your GP or menopause specialist is a great first step. When deciding to take HRT, each woman's risk versus benefit ratio needs to be understood. I am not a medical doctor. The domain of prescribing hormones falls to the medical profession. However, as a believer in knowledge is power, the more information women have before visiting their GP, the more successful the outcome for all.

I suggest that women print out a symptom checker, check off their symptoms, and bring it along to their doctor. This helps open the conversation and talk about the different formulations of use.

Why Choose HRT?

- If you have unmanageable or uncontrollable symptoms.
- If you have a challenging lifestyle with many demands.

- If you are not sleeping, feeling exhausted, or waking up drenched night after night.
- If early menopause begins before the age of 40 in order to protect your heart and bones.
- If symptoms are impacting on your relationships with your partner, children, or work colleagues.
- If you have low libido or vaginal dryness.
- To include it as a part of your preventative healthcare toolkit.
- To prevent osteoporosis, which is a bone disease women are at risk of as our oestrogen levels decrease. HRT is considered a buffer to maintaining bone density and preventing fractures.

If you are suffering from the above, become informed. It is worth giving HRT a trial as the benefits are likely to outweigh the risks.

Types of HRT

Here is a brief overview of the different formulations of HRT. Discuss with your doctor, and they will help you decide which option is right for you.

- *Systemic body-identical HRT* comes in tablet format, as a gel, patch, or spray.
- *Oestrogen-only HRT* is prescribed if your womb is removed (hysterectomy). There is no need for progesterone in this instance. Oestrogen-only HRT is associated with lower rates of breast cancer per 1,000 in women aged 50-59.
- *Combined HRT* if you have your womb, includes oestrogen and progesterone and is prescribed as a tablet, gel patch,

or spray. Micronised progesterone tablets and body identical oestrogen in patch gel or spray formulations are considered to have the least side effects. If you have a Mirena coil in situ for contraception, this contains localised progesterone, so you will only need oestrogen.

- *Vaginal oestrogen* in a pessary, gel, ring, or cream is prescribed for repeated urinary tract infections, dry vagina, or vulvovaginal atrophy. This may be prescribed with systemic HRT.

- *Testosterone* is available as a gel or implant.

What must be mentioned here is that HRT is not a panacea to menopausal symptoms. A whole of body approach deciding to prioritise your health when you reach perimenopause is going to enable you to thrive as you move through these years. HRT and other medications should be considered an add-on to your SOS toolkit, including lifestyle changes, nutrition, movement, and mindset work. The more options available in assisting women in navigating their menopause years, the better it is for all.

CHAPTER 21

MY STORY

"We cannot solve a problem we cannot see;
Thus, the need for public discourse to enable change."

\- Breeda Bermingham

By the time I had reached my 25th birthday, I had survived three car accidents, lost one of my closest and dearest friends Maura who died at age 22 from complications of a bone marrow transplant, and met my future husband John, father of our four children. Apart from this, the first part of my life was rather uneventful. Having been a mother for the past 27 years, along with working with mothers for many years, I feel mothers are truly awesome, with those parenting alone being "Olympians" in this world, constantly "spinning many plates in the air". I know and have met so many "lionesses" who would do anything for their children no matter what adversity they were facing in their own lives. Following the birth of our fourth child, Will, I stayed at home for ten years, returning to college to study psychology at age 49. When I was starting college, menopause was the furthest subject from my mind. It was not on my radar. I associated the cessation of my period with menopause full stop. As menopause is a retrospective diagnosis, many of us are right in the middle of this transition before understanding what is happening. No preparation, education, or openly available information contributes to this.

Is It Hot in Here, Or Is It Me?

Standing in the bar, chatting with friends at Listowel Races in September 2017, a ferocious heat gushed up my back, neck, face, forehead. My senses awakened. Beads of sweat dripped from the back of my neck. I uneasily peeled off my sunflower-colored jacket hoping to cool down, wondering if it was a result of the glass of white wine I had just tasted. Moving outdoors to watch the next race provided a wonderful distraction, and the cold autumn day provided a welcome release. I did not realise on that day at the races that this was the first flush of menopause.

Moving forward to the end of July 2018, as I sat under a sun lounger on Myrtle Beach, the smell of the salty sea clinging to my skin, feeling sorry for myself watching all around me swimming and splashing, another significant event was occurring. Feeling tired and irritable, massaging my crampy stomach under the windswept lounger, I was unaware that this was my last period. The last time I would have a monthly bleed, the end of my reproductive life. A massive landmark in a woman's life, yet unacknowledged in western culture. Looking back, I am delighted that this occurred during a magnificent three-week road trip in the United States with my sister, Eileen, and family. I am grateful for the fact that it remains so vivid as a great marker event. I reached menopause officially on the 31st of July 2019, one year after I had my last period.

Perimenopause had crept up on me. In the final year of college, I decided to start researching midlife women. Menopause is an integral part of this life stage. The word perimenopause was new to me, and the fact that it can last from two to eight years and be associated with 34 plus different symptoms was also a shocking revelation. I now understand why I was so angry when reviewing the research. There is a massive injustice to women in not understanding what is happening to us during perimenopause and menopause.

Understanding ourselves and accessing the correct support to manage severe symptoms is important to enable us to move through these years positively. This is key. Yes, there are lots of physical symptoms with many options from lifestyle, alternative therapies, and hormone replacement to help alleviate these. But it is pivotal to understand that there are emotional and psychological changes also occurring within at this time in life. Really listening to ourselves, enables us to find answers that work. Yoga, meditation, prayer, journaling are means of assisting us connect within. Doing the inner work helps reduce anxiety and low mood. I have always been someone who believes in the wisdom of the body. This really increased when our fourth Will was born at home. If we listen, there is much intelligence. It's about empowering ourselves to trust ourselves.

Interestingly, my story is that once my periods stopped, physical symptoms started arriving hot and heavy. Body odor, fluid retention, weight gain around the middle, irritability, tiredness, low energy, and rage or anger like I had not experienced before. Many women experience lots of symptoms before their last period, often in their early 40s. Every woman is different.

I consider myself well balanced in general. I try not to let things bother me, but this deep-seated anger was emerging. I was fortunate that in having become a menopause detective, I had seen the narrative of anger in the literature, so I knew it could be associated with our menopause journey. For me, it lasted approximately nine months, and the awareness of it enabled me to sit with it. A word of warning, the people closest to you are the ones who bear the brunt of this angry phase but be reassured it is only a phase, part of the transformation that is occurring within us at this time. There are many theories about rage, anger, and depression. Having navigated this journey with the above symptoms, I believe that anger enables us to get deeply in touch with who we are as women and access a deeper, more creative version of ourselves. There is something revelatory about it. I journaled a lot at this time, which was of great benefit, and I started to spend more and more time out in nature which started with Newstalk's Dr Ciara Kelly's *100 Days of Walking*. It was a time of reflection on life and gratitude. Everything comes up for review under a microscope – relationships, work, contribution. Giving ourselves permission to take this time and allow ourselves space is transformative and healing. I now realise this as I look back. Radical self-care does enable us to take on menopause. Fear and denial prolong symptoms.

I managed the physical symptoms, which lasted over two years, with lifestyle and food modifications. I got outside more, walked mindfully, played tennis three times a week, usually at 8 or 9 pm, prioritised self-care, and used supplements. I had gained a lot of weight which I found difficult to shift. I discovered Cortisol (stress hormone) was the hormone I needed to manage, and once I did, with the above modifications and occasional intermittent fasting, my symptoms settled. Many women find hormone replacement beneficial. I did not have sleep issues, night sweats, or constant flushes impacting my workday. If I did, I would probably have tried HRT. Red clover is a phytoestrogen and a natural replacement for those who may not wish to take or cannot take HRT. My belief is life is too short to suffer unnecessarily. Having turned 55 this year with a family history of osteoporosis, I have started to include body identical HRT (gel and micronized oral progesterone) in my preventative healthcare SOS toolkit along with weight-bearing exercise, Vitamin D, calcium, and DEXA screening. There is much evidence to support oestrogen replacement and optimal bone health.

I have discovered that managing menopause is all about empowering ourselves with information and finding what works for us. There is no one template that fits all. The problem to date is a lack of widely available information, no preparation, and little conversation. The taboo must be shattered for all women to have the support they deserve. Every woman is unique. As a menopause coach, I have found working in collaboration with women and creating individualised management plans creates the most successful outcomes. Women have a wonderful, innate ability to choose what is right for them once provided with information and education. Using the analogy of menopause as a bridge that all women cross over, albeit rocky and turbulent at times, assists women in understanding this is a transition, one that can be controlled and navigated with support. Many of us need help getting over the bridge. Opening the conversation and smashing the taboo will enable more of us to do so successfully and thrive.

I refer to much of Part Four in our six-week courses and coaching programs which are facilitated in groups or individually. If we succeed in normalising the conversation around menopause in society, talking as we do about pregnancy, women are given the opportunity to seize this exciting stage of their lives. Girls and women should be educated early about this phase of life, with the focus shifting from the old negative to the newer, more positive story, thereby helping demystify the taboo, reducing fear, silence, and shame.

- The question we all need to ask is who benefits from a new story?
- What impact societally and culturally would a new story on menopause have?
- What happens if we choose to accept the status quo and blindly continue to remain quiet?

I believe when women get together, anything is possible. Language is powerful, and words change and transform. I include here a synopsis of two stories in the research literature. The old has been given precedence for years and has overshadowed the newer version. It is time the world saw these two stories. You decide which will benefit women.

PART FIVE

AMAZING ADVOCATES WORKING IN "MENOPAUSE-LAND"

CHAPTER 22

THE CHANGEMAKERS

"When we change the way we look at things the things,
we look at change"

- Dr Wayne Dyer

Over the past two to three years, an increasing number
of midlife women are emerging onto public platforms
to talk openly about menopause for the first time in
history, offering support to other women. This is how we will
break down the power of taboo. Taboos thrive in silence, with
societal and generational change occurring slowly. Although
disrupting the status quo is challenging, it can be done! I am a
huge believer in the power of collaboration. By getting together
and amplifying our voice around menopause, we will engage
governments and health departments who will realise that
menopause is a highly significant transition in a woman's life
and needs to be recognised.

Within this part of *Midlife Women Rock* are the voices of
trailblazing women (and one man), who I have come to know
both in the United Kingdom and Ireland. They are advocates for
change as well as supporting and empowering women to take on
their menopause years with zest.

Sam Palmer, a trailblazer in the menopause arena, is passionate about getting women moving at menopause. She is a former nurse who focuses on the benefits of movement as medicine and how it impacts women's physical and mental health. Sam and I met at Meg Mathews menopause conference in London in 2019. She can be found at www.midlifemakeover.com

Nicki Williams is an award-winning nutritionist, author, and speaker who has worked with 1,000's of women in the United Kingdom and Ireland. A regular contributor to media, she is passionate about women accessing support during perimenopause and menopause. I worked alongside Nicki at the trailblazing *Embrace* three-day event on menopause in October 2020. A lot of her work revolves around educating women on the fact that we have many hormones in our bodies. The "Feisty Four" - cortisol, insulin, oestrogen, and progesterone - are Nicki's favourite. Nicki is at www.happyhormonesforlife.com

Lorraine Boyce from County Donegal, is a pelvic floor physiotherapist and founder of *Down Below Physio*. Her passion is pelvic floor health. She is on a mission to highlight that help is available to women with pelvic floor, urinary, and vaginal issues which emerge during perimenopause and menopause. It is never too late to start investing in your pelvic health. We just need to open the conversation more. Lorraine and I are both contributors to the Women's Taskforce on menopause in Ireland. Lorraine can be found at www.downbelowphysio.ie

Suné Markowitz-Shulman from Oxford participated in the wonderful *Embrace Menopause and Midlife* three-day event in October 2020. Suné works with women in menopause, helping them slow down and find peace within. Mindfulness is another tool to consider adding to our SOS toolbox. Slowing down our life is transformative if symptoms are debilitating and impacting our mental health. Suné can be found at www.simplysune.com

Dr Mary Ryan is a consultant endocrinologist and menopause advocate from Limerick. Having worked with 1000's of women navigating different stages of menopause, she provides her top tips for navigating this life transition. Mary is a well-known media spokesperson and has contributed widely on the empowerment of women, a subject she is passionate about. She has been delighted to see the increased interest in opening the conversation around menopause in Ireland in recent years. Mary and I met at the *Vitality Expo* in 2019. She has a regular podcast and can be found at www.drmaryryan.com

Ilona Madden is a nutritional therapist and coach from Bray, Co Wicklow. She is also a speaker at the *Midlife Women Rock Café*. Ilona is passionate about helping busy women who want to get their energy back, get their "crazy" hormones under control, and feel like their "old" self again. She says she is living proof that one can be fitter and stronger in midlife with diet and lifestyle changes. Here, she shares her top tips from working with women. She can be found at www.rightfood4u.ie_

Dinah Siman is a Pilates instructor and menopause advocate. Dinah is another powerful trailblazer wanting to ensure women understand the power of Pilates, posture, and strengthening our core and pelvic floor as we move through menopause. Her popular videos on Instagram have 1000's following her weekly tips on positively managing the change. Follow Dinah at @ *menopausepilates* on Instagram.

Dr Mark Rowe is a GP, author, and a sought after expert in positive health and lifestyle medicine. He aims to help us answer the question, "How can we live more vitally?" At the core of his practice, he understands that to improve our physical health, we also need to consider our mindset, our mental wellbeing and purpose. An advocate for women, he champions us to reap the benefits from positive change. He can be found at www. drmarkrowe.com. His popular podcast In the DOCTOR'S CHAIR has 1,000's of subscribers and can be found on Apple Spotify and on his website.

CHAPTER 23

SAM PALMER:
MOVEMENT AS MEDICINE

Wh…en you haven't slept, have joints that ache when you move, and the thought of pouring yourself into lycra makes you shudder, it's hard to embrace the fact that movement is medicine for women in perimenopause and beyond. But here's the thing, as oestrogen declines, even the most ardent gym-goer in a previous life will be at risk of thinning bones, muscle loss, and an increased risk of heart disease unless steps are taken to avoid it.

Whether a woman chooses to take HRT or not, to stay mobile, healthy, and vibrant in menopause and beyond, movement becomes a non-negotiable, just like cleaning our teeth. The right type of exercise will ease sore joints, improve sleep, stabilise mood swings and help with weight control. So why don't we see midlife women queuing up outside gyms and desperate to join online fitness classes?

In my opinion, very few fitness instructors understand what women need at this time, nor do they plan workouts with our menopausal body in mind. We don't need endurance workouts with an instructor shouting commands to perform exercises designed for men twenty years younger than us.

Nor do we need classes that focus on "getting ripped," which often put huge pressure on an already compromised pelvic floor (once again, oestrogen is at play here) and lead to such exhaustion that we need to lie down for the afternoon. Instead, we should focus on having a varied tool kit of exercise focusing on these areas:

- **Strength** is a new type of workout for many midlife women and often the one they are most daunted by. Exercise which involves lifting your own body weight, or dumbbells, resistance bands, or even domestic heavy objects, is vital. It helps redress muscle loss and bone thinning, which occur as part of ageing. 20-30 minutes of this type of workout twice a week will reap physical and mental benefits.

- **Sweat.** Yes, we may be sweating more than is comfortable right now but sweating as a result of exercise means an increased heart rate which will help to reduce the risk of heart disease. Even a simple walk can be turned into a cardio workout by swinging your arms and increasing your pace and going uphill. Of course, we can sweat cycling, running, dancing, and even doing gardening or other manual chores.

- **Slow.** Many of us find this the hardest type of movement to incorporate because we don't see its value in terms of exercise. The aim of slow movement is to find some calm inside a frantic brain and to switch off cortisol production. Traditionally, yoga is a perfect way to do this, but you may enjoy a stroll through a forest, a leisurely cycle along the coast, or perhaps a relaxing freestyle dance.

The best exercise is the one you love because you will continue to do it, but be mindful of including **Strength, Sweat, and Something Slow** where you can.

CHAPTER 24

NICKI WILLIAMS: HAPPY HORMONES FOR LIFE

It is wonderful to see more and more women investing in their health and wellbeing. Having worked with many women navigating different stages of menopause, here are my top tips.

Self-Care Is Non-negotiable

If stress is the number one hormone disruptor, then this is the time to make self-care a non-negotiable in your life. That means prioritising your needs over and above everything and everyone. Take more time for yourself, slow down, listen to your needs, and make sure they are being met. You've probably never done this before if you've spent your life looking after others, but this is your time. Make sure you do this, and you'll have a much better quality of life during and beyond menopause.

Menopause Affects Your Mental Health

We know about the physical symptoms – hot flushes, night sweats, fatigue, mood swings, PMS, etc. But changing hormones can also affect the brain and have a big impact on your mental health. Common symptoms include depression, anxiety, mood swings, emotions, brain fog, low motivation, lack of focus, and memory loss.

Your Diet Matters (a Lot!)

What you eat during this phase of your life matters more than ever. This is the time to start nourishing yourself with the right foods. Nutrients that support your hormones and don't disrupt them. No more dieting, calorie counting, or limiting fat (the good kind). Your hormones will thank you!

Stress Matters Even More

I used to think it was your diet that was more important (I am a nutritionist after all), but now after supporting so many women over the years, I really do believe that stress is the number one indicator of how good or bad your menopause journey will be. When cortisol and adrenaline become elevated for long periods burnout follows.

HRT Is Not the Only Option

I love HRT when it's needed. However, standard treatments are only ever going to replace two or three of your hormones (oestrogen, progesterone, testosterone). You have so many other hormones that could be out of balance, including (cortisol, insulin, thyroid), so HRT has its limitations, and it won't always work for everyone (or you may not be able or want to take it).

Perimenopause Can Start in Your 30s!

This is when your eggs start to run out, and your hormones start to change. But you might not notice any symptoms until your mid to late 40s. The earlier you can prepare for perimenopause, the better journey you're likely to have.

Testing Can Provide the Missing Link

Hormone testing isn't that reliable (or helpful) when you're doing blood tests. But state of the art urine tests for hormones can be a game-changer. If you want to dig deeper and find out what your hormones are actually up to, these tests are extremely valuable.

The Right Type of HRT Is Safe (And Natural)

HRT has come a long way since the shocking study in 2002 highlighting its risks and side effects. Those studies (and subsequent ones) were done on synthetic forms of oestrogen and progesterone. Nowadays, we have access to body-identical HRT, which is molecularly identical to your own hormones, making it a safe and natural way to replace your hormones.

There Is No One Size Fits All Treatment

Menopause is often seen as a "problem" that clearly there must be a "fix" for. The problem is that every woman is unique. We have different genes, biochemistries, lifestyles, diets, stresses, histories, beliefs, and environments. Every woman deserves to make an informed choice and decide what's right for her (no judgement).

Menopause Can Be the Best Thing to Happen to You!

OK, bear with me on this one! Menopause marks a precious time in your life. You're heading into the second phase of your life. It can actually be liberating. You can experience a kind of freedom, from caring what others think (thank you, Helen Mirren!), to being more yourself than you've ever been. It can be the catalyst to a new you and a new life - something to be embraced.

CHAPTER 25

LORRAINE BOYCE: DOWN BELOW PHYSIO

I was a musculoskeletal physiotherapist for years, but I realised my passion and interest was really in pelvic health. I wanted to help women with their pelvic floor issues, so I made it the sole focus of my clinical practice and changed my business name to *Down Below Physio!* And yes, it does exactly what it says on the tin; I do physio for your 'down below' area. So many women still don't realise that there are physiotherapists who specialise in this area of health, and it's my mission to let women know that there is help available. One benefit that has come out of the pandemic is that it is more accessible than ever to access services, with virtual consultations becoming more commonplace. Even if you don't have a dedicated pelvic health physiotherapy clinic near you, you can still find help online.

I treat bladder and bowel issues, such as urgency, frequency, incontinence, and constipation. I treat pelvic organ prolapse, pelvic pain patterns, and abdominal muscle separation. I treat women in pregnancy and do postnatal 'mummy check-ups' afterwards. I help women with painful sex, penetration issues, and vaginal dryness.

When we think about self-care, what often springs to mind is a bubble bath, a face mask, and a glass of wine, which of course is lovely, but I think there's no better, more practical form of self-care than prioritising yourself by making an appointment to take care of your pelvic health. Unattended to symptoms can affect you mentally and emotionally. They can affect your confidence, your intimate relationship, and your ability to work or exercise. Women attending my clinic have time to talk and share in a private, supportive environment. It's incredibly important for women to feel informed and supported as they experience changes in perimenopause and menopause, including changes in pelvic health.

As oestrogen levels decline in menopause, it can affect vaginal, vulvar, urinary, and rectal tissues. The range of symptoms you can experience as a result is known as 'Genitourinary Syndrome of Menopause' or GSM. There is evidence to show that this affects many women, yet only 7% receive treatment. That's why it's so important to get the message out there that clinics like my own here at *Down Below Physio* exist.

With menopause, your vulvo-vaginal tissues can become thinner, drier, and less able to adapt to stretch. They may feel itchy, irritated, or inflamed, and sex can become painful or impossible. You may experience recurrent urinary tract infections, urinary urgency, frequency or leaking. The sphincter of your bowel may be affected, and you may not be able to keep in gas or stool.

But before this becomes very depressing, these symptoms respond really well to physiotherapy, exercises, and localised hormonal treatment. Investing in yourself is key.

My Top Tips for Your Pelvic Floor

- Sometimes we don't think of our pelvic floor until we're getting symptoms, but pelvic floor exercises are for everyone and for life.

- A 'down below' check-up can help you understand what's happening and what you need to do to improve your symptoms. Expert advice and support are available.

- And most importantly, while these symptoms are all very common, they don't have to be 'normal' or something that you just put up with. Make sure to take care of and invest in yourself 'down below.'

CHAPTER 26

SUNÉ MARKOWITZ-SHULMAN: MINDFUL MENOPAUSE

Midlife and menopause create beautiful and meaningful moments to reflect on – growing families, self-confidence, maturity, friendships, professional accomplishments – the list is endless, but for many of us, the physical and psychological changes and symptoms can be so overwhelming that it feels like we are being swept away by an uncontrollable storm. Many women feel like they lose themselves, hardly recognising this woman they have become. It does not have to be this way.

Jon Kabat Zinn, one of the founding fathers, defines mindfulness as "paying attention in a particular way: on purpose, in the present moment and non-judgmentally." All of us can do this, and all of us can find ways to do it more. It is not reserved for the privileged. You do not need to sit on a mountain top to meditate, and there is no special state to reach.

This means that it's never too late, and you are never too old to start practicing mindfulness and realise the benefits for your midlife, menopause, and beyond.

Most of our lives are spent on autopilot, going through the motions of our day from morning to night in trance-like routines. We pride ourselves on multitasking, being busy, stressed, and pay trivial attention to the details of our inner and outer lives. For many of us, until a momentous event (like menopause) happens, we take little time to pause and reflect. Mindfulness helps us to do exactly that; pause, observe and reflect, regularly. Instead of reacting to every emotional or physical state we find ourselves in (which we may or may not be aware of), mindfulness offers breathing space and perspective, creating a moment to choose so that we can act with calmness and intent.

Mindfulness may not make our symptoms or wrinkles disappear, but it can help cultivate a different relationship to our changing bodies and selves. It helps us to orientate towards attitudes of patience, self-compassion, acceptance, kindness, trust, non-judgement, and gratitude.

Instead of viewing changes with regret or longing for past ideals, mindfulness helps us be more aware of our thoughts, emotions, bodily sensations, and impulses and to move closer to what is already here with curiosity and kindness instead of pushing it away or ignoring it.

We may succumb to quick fixes that help in the short-term, but tomorrow when the sleeping pills have worn off, the whole chocolate cake has been eaten, and every cup has been thrown against a wall because of uncontrollable rage, we are still feeling angry, hot, and unheard.

Mindfulness teaches us acceptance, which is not the same as giving up. It helps us to let go of the urge to fix or change the things that we can't and to approach life and all its beauty and suffering with openness, awareness, and kindness. It helps us notice feelings of anxiety and frustration and cultivate gratitude for the mundane. Yes, that includes hot flushes, changing moods, and sleepless nights, but because we are also cultivating self-compassion and empowerment, we may just learn to appreciate and understand our worth and reach out for help. Not because we're weak or useless, but because we are stronger in mind, body, and spirit!

Important side note: Mindfulness is not a panacea or a cure. It's a tool that can help lots of people live healthier, happier, and more fulfilled lives. This is especially important to remember for people who have previous trauma or have serious mental health conditions. Mindfulness should not take the place of therapy in these cases and should be practiced with a registered and trained mindfulness teacher who is also trauma-informed.

CHAPTER 27

Dr MARY RYAN: NAVIGATING THE MENOPAUSE YEARS

Having worked with women at various stages of menopause for years, here are my top recommendations.

Top Tips for Navigating Your Menopause Years:

1. Education is key. Know the symptoms. There are 34 plus.

2. Listen to your body. For years women have not fully understood the power of their bodies. We have much wisdom.

3. Rest is vital if symptoms are bad. Don't try to push through. And drop the guilt.

4. Eat healthy and reduce caffeine.

5. Take natural supplements, including magnesium, B complex, and Vitamin D. *Clean Marine MenoMin* is a good brand.

6. Pelvic floor exercises are a must as oestrogen depletion affects the pelvic floor muscles. It is never too late to start.

7. Hormone replacement therapy is also available as long as it suits you and you do not have a family history of ovarian, breast, or uterine cancer. Discuss with your doctor.

8. Oestrogen pessaries are available for vaginal dryness.

9. Medications are available for peripheral neuropathy and restless leg. Talk to your GP.

10. There is much help available. Reach out. No woman needs to suffer in silence.

CHAPTER 28

ILONA MADDEN: BALANCING FOOD in MIDLIFE

A s our bodies change, our requirements for nutrients change, and it's important to adapt to those changes and not say, "But I used to be able to eat…" The main focus when it comes to nutrition is to add nutrients, especially those that naturally decline with age, and to avoid adding foods that put pressure on our systems.

Balance Your Blood Sugar

As we age and our hormones change, our bodies become more sensitive to insulin, and therefore, one of the most important things to do is to reduce the amount of sugars and carbohydrates in your diet. It's not just about eating sweets and desserts, but also about all the hidden sugars in ready-made sauces and products (hence cooking from scratch).

Eat More Vegetables and a Higher Variety of Vegetables

We all know eating vegetables is important, but did you know:

- Fibre keeps you fuller for longer.

- Each colour vegetable feeds various bacteria in your gut. These, in turn, will look after your mood, your immune system, and even your weight.

- Vegetables contain a huge variety of nutrients, minerals, vitamins, and phytonutrients which all help our bodies function the way they're designed to.

- They are important for detoxification and elimination. Hormonal imbalance can happen when hormones are "recycled" instead of being "eliminated."

- If you don't like vegetables, it is usually because you haven't prepared them properly so far. There are so many vegetables out there. Nobody can say they do not like all of them!

Phytoestrogens

These are substances that can sit on the oestrogen receptors in your body, i.e., mimicking the function of the oestrogen hormone, and therefore potentially lessen some of the symptoms that come from a reduction in oestrogen. The best sources of phytoestrogens are soy products (make sure it's not genetically modified and preferably fermented), nuts and seeds, especially flaxseeds, and legumes.

Anti-Inflammatory Foods

Low-grade inflammation in our bodies is the cause of many of our modern health issues, such as heart disease, diabetes, Alzheimer's, and joint pain. Omega 3 is one of the most important anti-inflammatory agents. You will find it in oily fish, such as salmon and mackerel. Ginger, turmeric, and garlic are the best spices and should be added to all dishes.

Foods That Support Liver Detoxification

In order to keep our hormones balanced, it is equally important to make sure detoxification is working optimally. Certain foods and herbs help support the detoxification: lemon and warm water; red onions; garlic; green leafy vegetables; cruciferous vegetables; eggs; beef; oysters (zinc); bitter vegetables and herbs; beetroot; nettle.

Healthy Fats

Fats have been demonised for so long, but all our cells have fat around them. Our brain is made up of fat, and cholesterol is a vital substance to keep us alive. For our neurotransmitters and hormones, it is vital to get adequate fat in your diet. Also, fat is important to absorb our fat-soluble vitamins such as Vitamin A, E, and D (which in turn is important for the bones). Avocados, extra virgin olive oil, olives, coconut oil, nuts, and seeds are good sources of healthy fats.

Calcium

Calcium is important for our bones, but without the right nutrients to make it absorbable, there is no point in adding it to the diet, whether in food or supplement form. Vitamin D, vitamin K, magnesium, boron, zinc, and B-vitamins are all needed. You'll get all of this with a balanced diet. For bone building, you also need to make collagen, and for that, you need plenty of vitamin C. Sesame seeds are also high in calcium.

Intermittent Fasting

When we fast, our body has time to rest, digest, and heal. I recommend starting with 12 hours of not eating, which is quite easy to do when finishing your dinner at 7 pm. Just don't have your breakfast before 7 am. Gradually build up to 14 or 16 hours. The main benefit apart from being in "repair" mode is that it also improves your insulin resistance and helps tap into fat-burning mode.

CHAPTER 29

DINAH SIMAN:
PILATES FOR MENOPAUSE

Why choose Pilates for menopause, fitness, and wellbeing?

Menopause Pilates is my passion project. I've taught women in menopause for over 23 years, and of course, there's nothing like your own experience to transform knowledge into wisdom. I am a post-menopausal woman. I consider myself incredibly blessed that I was introduced to Pilates in my early 30s. It's been my go-to exercise method ever since.

I've never been sporty, but I've always loved movement. So much so that in addition to teaching Pilates, I'm qualified to teach Franklin Method, Gyrotonic® and yoga as well as exercise to music. But it is Pilates that has supported me through my menopause transition. It is uniquely suited to our menopausal body.

We know that movement is vital for our health and wellbeing during the stages of menopause. Hormonal depletion reduces our muscle mass, can precipitate osteoporosis, slows our healing from injury, and can increase inflammatory pain in joints and soft tissue. We're often sleep-deprived and anxious, and our metabolism may be under siege, with unwelcome weight gain. It's so crucial we understand that we may have to adjust the way we exercise and address the needs of our changing body. In my experience, this can be an incredibly empowering and rejuvenating time of possibilities - we just need to listen to our body and respond with self-care, compassion, and the appropriate movement practice.

Pilates is a method of exercise that works our whole system. Strength and resistance exercise, either on the mat using your own body weight and small props such as bands or in the Pilates studio on the large spring-based equipment, are key to the method. Bone loading movements are inherent in the practice, balance, stability, core strength, and attention to breathing. The understanding of breathwork enhances the focus on pelvic floor health, ensuring participants recognise the need to release as well as engage pelvic floor muscles. Pilates practice ensures appropriate spinal movement to counter the postural issues we may encounter from too much sitting and driving. There is a gentle but consistent reminder in Pilates to tune into your body awareness, observe how your body is feeling with no judgement, and enjoy nutritious movements. These nurture and support our system, reduce stress and promote the confidence that we can support ourselves.

Many women lose the confidence to go to a gym or an exercise class. Some totally lose the joy of moving. Pilates is the perfect route back to fitness and an enhanced understanding of how to move your body with ease. During perimenopause, I had to completely overhaul my exercise. Inflammatory pain and symptoms of hypermobility increased as my hormones depleted. My knowledge and practice of Pilates instinctively enabled me to bed down into the micro-movements I needed to support my body, gradually enabling me to increase my strength and stability. I had to abandon all my other movement practices. Pilates is the balanced path in exercise for me. It gives such strong foundations for safe, supportive, and positive movement practice.

CHAPTER 30

DR MARK ROWE: MIDLIFE - CRISIS OR OPPORTUNITY?

Ⓞ ne of the recurring themes in my podcast conversations, *In the Doctors Chair*, is how to recharge from stress and build a more resilient mind. Middle-aged people, in particular, are more stressed than ever before, perhaps experiencing up to 19% more stress now than two decades ago (equating to an extra 64 days of stress each year), according to research from Penn State University.

For women reaching midlife, stressors arise from differing sources. Concurrent demands from growing family or empty nest, elderly parents, concern about health, traumatic life events such as the death of a loved one, divorce, loss of fertility, or financial concerns, may result in a persistent sense of grief, pining for the past and challenging your sense of who you are. Add in the general sense of life "speeding up," smartphone distraction, and the backdrop of a continuous news cycle. On top of that, the growing obsession with staying young, played out on social media, can place more pressure to paper over the cracks of advancing age.

Little wonder the term "midlife crisis" can raise its head, even before you consider the impact of menopause with its physiologically changing hormone levels, as stress is a huge hormone disruptor.

This is why self-care during the menopause years should be a priority. As a doctor, I believe health is priceless, the greatest gift there is - the crown on the well person's head that only the sick person can see. Taking good care of yourself is a key strategy to recover and recharge from life stress as well as for self-renewal and a life of vitality. Unfortunately, self-care is often one of the first things to fall by the wayside in times of stress.

One of the great paradoxes about self-care is that people can be so generous towards others and yet so miserly and severe when it comes to giving themselves some slack. You can't pour from an empty cup. Self-care gives you the energy and capacity to give more to others.

Research from Dr Christakis at Yale University has found that emotional positivity spreads outwards to three degrees of separation through your social networks, impacting your friends and their friends.

The best and most impactful forms of self-care are simple, inexpensive, and don't take much time, which brings me to mindfulness and meditation. Both practices support self-care through the cultivation of awareness and attention.

I have developed a mindful technique that I call "PAUSE" - to consciously slow your breathing down to four or five breaths per minute. Check it out on my website www.drmarkrowe.com

Mindful breathing dampens the stress centre or red button in the brain (amygdala), decreases feelings of anxiety, negative stress, and brain fog, building emotional calm and contentment. It is a terrific reminder that you are in control.

Mindful breathing has to be one of the simplest and most effective habits to enhance your overall vitality and enabling you to connect with your spirit and purpose. Try it and see for yourself.

There are many strategies to support your wellbeing in midlife. Focus on the little things you can control, protect your sleep, exercise, and move regularly, eat good food, spend time in nature, and build strong supportive relationships. If you're struggling, remember it's good to talk. Consider talking to your doctor, to a trained therapist (CBT, therapy can be invaluable), to a coach, or to your friends. You can gain fresh perspectives.

A study published in the *International Journal of Behavioural Development* has found that experiencing a "crisis" (whether at midlife or earlier) enhanced participants curiosity about themselves and the wider world around them, supporting creativity, growth, and new ways of being in the world, moving the conversation from, "What have I lost?" to "How I can grow?"

The Chinese symbol for crisis also means opportunity. Our midlife years can be a great opportunity to reconnect with the essence of who you are, rediscover your purpose, and embrace a mindset of growth and possibility. To live with more vitality and to never stop starting. What are you waiting for?

CONCLUSION:

BOLDLY MOVING FORWARD

Menopause is a highly significant individual experience that women globally transition through. The narratives to date expose a massive absence in preparation, education, information, and understanding of this life transition. We each arrive at perimenopause with our own history, genetic makeup, perspectives, and opinions. Looking at menopause macroscopically, the stereotypical characterisation of menopausal women persists because the taboo has kept women silenced. Remaining silent is the enemy and has ongoing consequences for women's wellbeing. There is no longer a legitimacy in constructing menopause as an overwhelmingly negative life stage. Past generations accepted invisibility; we have a choice now. Opening conversation and normalising discourse around this life stage is key to shifting perspectives and creating a new story for a new generation of midlife women.

As life expectancy increases, women are likely to have more adult years post-menopause than before. Consider for a minute that you are sitting on a rocking chair at age 90, looking back at your midlife years. Did you ensure your health and wellbeing were a priority? Investing in you is an investment in all your relationships. It helps reduce stress levels, prevent disease, and increases your wellbeing. A win-win all around. What possibilities do you see? What would you like to try now that you may have more time for? We need to open ourselves up to the potentials and possibilities that this phase of life brings. The doom and gloom rhetoric has kept too many too quiet and feeling as though the best of life is over.

How we eat, move, sleep and think (positive or negative) during menopause is directly associated with us surviving or thriving. We have the power to find what will best help us navigate these years. Keep remembering you are worth it.

I like the idea of blue-sky thinking, creatively looking at things in completely new ways. The time has come to apply some of the principles to the framing and characterisation of menopause, both culturally and in everyday society. Having silenced us for decades, the taboo must be lifted to best serve women transitioning through these years. The depictions of women in menopause must be challenged. A re characterisation of what a menopausal woman looks and feels like is needed and called for by many women. Every public conversation you have about menopause is a step closer to ensuring the discourse surrounding this phase of life becomes mainstream. In doing so, we increase public traction and funding, leading to increased supports for those who need them. Women will be the changemakers here if we work collaboratively raising other women up along the way.

What motivated me to start working in Menopause-Land was the massive injustice to women, families, and society that has been allowed to continue due to silence and deficiencies in education and support. When women are isolated from one another and suffering in silence, they cannot create change as they have no voice. Mute women and shame have been synonymous with menopause. However, in the cafés, I have witnessed narratives change when women come together, share stories, support one another in tears and laughter. Women access their voice and agency. As more and more women come together, speak up about menopause, advocate for supports, we bring about necessary cultural change. This is how we shift perspectives. Fully functioning progressive societies depend upon inclusion, and inclusion means recognising the value as well as the needs of menopausal women.

We need to have the courage to call out and question the prevailing cultural norms that hide the bias against menopausal women. If enough of us call it out, things can change. Once we bring this into the public domain, more and more women and men will see the scandal that has existed for decades and stand against it. This is how we expose social norms that hide the bias we are blind to. When we see them, we end them. Rolling out the nationwide education and awareness campaign committed to by the Irish government and Department of Health will see Ireland as the first country in the world to instigate such a campaign and will hopefully encourage other countries to follow.

In reading this book, I hope you got an overview of how, in 2021, we are where we are in Menopause-Land. Educating and empowering oneself on menopause, understanding the four dimensions, and the availability of HRT, will dramatically impact how you experience this time of life. You have the power to thrive through this time once you manage symptoms.

Seismic change has occurred in the UK since I attended the Meg Mathews conference in May 2019, with Ireland starting to follow. Every day, women are using their voice, coming into this space, leading this change, and being supported by celebrities and politicians. It is up to us women to continue to advocate for necessary supports, in particular for younger women and in the workplace. The possibility of a new story for women as we move through this phase of life may accelerate in smashing the taboo. How can we all contribute to changing the narrative? Who wins if we shift the focus of the menopause story? Are we blindly holding onto the old story? Why? These are questions to reflect upon. Language is powerful. It can lift us up or knock and keep us down. We need to resist and challenge the overwhelming negative discourse. How is the present language surrounding failure, loss, deficiency, degeneration, and disease helping women? By focusing primarily on medicalising menopause, we miss the bigger picture, the importance of the **meaning** of this phase of life, and it is in women understanding this that empowerment begins, or they get their power back. Knowing you have the power to take control and manage your menopause can shift your mindset and attitudes. Our voices count. We are the fastest growing cohort of women in the workplace, and there is power in numbers. Stories have the power to change a culture. Menopause leads to new opportunities, second chances, access to a deep creative power, courage, a kick-ass attitude, and innate leadership. If you knew this lay ahead as you moved through this phase of life, would you still be fearful? Would you be in denial, ashamed, or silenced? Many women and men's voices are referred to in this book. To ignite cultural change we need a collaborative approach. I am an optimist by nature. I love seeking possibilities and potentials in others and in life. Continuing to amplify voices of many around the subject of menopause will creatively shift perspectives.

I wish you all the very best on your menopause journey. There is a valuable SOS toolkit provided within the pages of this book. The world needs the magnificent skillset you have acquired by midlife. For years, women have been leaders in their homes, juggling families, relationships, home management, and careers. Women often need to be reminded of how talented they are. Society would benefit greatly from more of these women emerging and becoming visible. We look at life through a different lens. I am not saying it is better. It is simply that we prioritise differently. Reach out for support if needed. You have the power now.

Please feel free to get in touch with me. Remember, we are opening and exploring this conversation together. Email me at breeda@midlifewomenrockproject.com.

Breeda is available to do podcast guesting workplace presentations and is a Keynote speaker.

MOVING FORWARD, PROVOKING CHANGE

There has been:

No Preparation to Date

We can change this with education in schools and colleges, GP and allied healthcare staff training. This is a public health issue. A preventative approach will work best here.

No Education to Date

This can change with governments and health departments recognising the need to educate all of society. With any new policy it's about prioritisation. Menopause was neglected for decades and needs showcasing. We must drop the shame.

The Irish government has committed to a nationwide campaign. Campaigns and programmes need to become widely available.

No Widely Accessible Information

Media can help here. We need to saturate popular culture with the new story on menopause as was done with pregnancy. Reduce the negative discourse. It has not helped women.

Magazines, newspapers, academia, business, tech can all become involved and interested in menopause. Stop focusing on the negative story. It is not helping women or society.

Quick Reference Guide

The Power of Language	
OLD STORY	**NEW STORY**
Loss	Opportunities
Crisis	Overcoming
Degeneration	Second Chances
Deficiency	Access To:
Crisis	Deep Creativity
Failure	Empowerment
Downhill	Courage
Devalued	Innate Leadership

Menopause encompasses an arena that is part of a much broader lack of understanding and a shortage of research into midlife women's life experiences. Unlike pregnancy and childbirth, every woman on the planet will experience menopause. Yet, to date, the universal story does not appear to respect its immense significance in a woman's lifespan.

In the 1990s, Dr Gail Sheedy, in writing *Silent Passage* (1998), attempted to open up the conversation. There is an excellent paragraph in her book in which she said when she appeared on the Oprah Winfrey show, the producer told her that it was easier booking guests who had murdered their spouses than finding women to talk about menopause. Another example of the power of taboo and suppression of women's voices.

Most Common Symptoms

Irregular periods

Hot flushes

Night sweats

Sleep disturbance

Loss of libido

Physical Symptoms

Weight gain

Irregular heartbeat or palpitations

Bladder problems

Hair loss

Tiredness or no energy

Dizziness

Body odour

Bloating

Brittle nails

Allergies

Osteopenia/Osteoporosis

Psychological Changes

Mood swings

Irritability

Anxiety

Poor concentration

Brain fog

Depression

Anger or rage

Other Symptoms

Headaches or migraine

Tinnitus

Breast pain

Joint pain

Burning mouth or tongue

Dental and gum issues

Dry and itchy skin

Muscle spasm

Digestive upsets

Tingling extremities

Electric shock

References

Introduction

Beard, M. (2017). *Women & power: a manifesto*. London: Liveright Publishing Corporation.

Brown, B. (2008). *I thought it was just me (but it isn't): making the journey from "What will people think?" to "I am enough."* New York: Avery.

Brown, B. (2018). *Dare to Lead: Brave Work. Tough Conversations. Whole Hearts*. London: Ebury Publishing.

Brown, L., Bowden, S., Bryant, C., Brown, V., Bei, B., Gilson, K.-M., Komiti, A. and Judd, F. (2015). Validation and utility of the Attitudes to Ageing Questionnaire: Links to menopause and well-being trajectories. *Maturitas*, 82(2), pp.190–196.

Brown, L., Bryant, C., Brown, V., Bei, B. and Judd, F. (2015). Investigating how menopausal factors and self-compassion shape well-being: An exploratory path analysis. *Maturitas*, 81(2), pp.293–299.

Cronin-Bermingham, B. (2020). *Silence Taboo and Midlife Women: A case study of the Midlife Women Rock Café in Waterford city* [Masters dissertation]. https://mural.maynoothuniversity.ie/14196/

DeAngelis, T. (2010). Menopause, the makeover: Psychologists are helping women sidestep the stereotypes associated with menopause and transform this developmental passage into a vital new phase of life. *American Psychological Association*, 41(3), pp. 40.

Jack, G., Pitts, M., Riach, K., Bariola, E., Schapper, J., & Sarrel, P. (2014). *Women, Work and the Menopause: Releasing the Potential of Older Professional Women.* https://womenworkandthemenopause.files.wordpress.com/2014/09/women-work-and-the-menopause-final-report.pdf

Jack, G., Riach, K., & Bariola, E. (2019). Temporality and gendered agency: Menopausal subjectivities in women's work. *Human Relations*, 72(1), pp. 122–143.

Lesser, E. (2022). *Cassandra Speaks: when women are the storytellers, the human story changes.* New York: Harper Wave.

Montero, G., de Montero, A., & de Vogelfanger, L. (Eds.). (2013). *Updating Midlife Psychoanalytic Perspectives.* Abingdon: Routledge.

OlaOlorun, F. M., & Shen, W. (2020). Menopause. *Oxford Research Encyclopedia of Global Public Health.* https://doi.org/10.1093/acrefore/9780190632366.013.176

Orth, U. and Robins, R.W. (2014). The Development of Self-Esteem. *Current Directions in Psychological Science*, [online] 23(5), pp.381–387. Available at: https://journals.sagepub.com/doi/10.1177/0963721414547414.

Orth, U., Robins, R.W., Trzesniewski, K.H., Maes, J. and Schmitt, M. (2009). Low self-esteem is a risk factor for depressive symptoms from young adulthood to old age. *Journal of Abnormal Psychology*, [online] 118(3), pp.472–478. Available at: https://uorth.files.wordpress.com/2010/08/orth_et_al_2009_jap.pdf.

Ussher, J.M., Hawkey, A.J. and Perz, J. (2018). "Age of despair", or "when life starts": migrant and refugee women negotiate constructions of menopause. *Culture, Health & Sexuality*, 21(7), pp.741–756.

WHO Scientific Group on Research on the Menopause in the 1990s (1994: Geneva, Switzerland), & World Health Organization. (1996). *Research on the menopause in the 1990s: report of a WHO scientific group.* https://apps.who.int/iris/handle/10665/41841

Chapter 1

Doyle, G. (2020). *Untamed.* New York: The Dial Press.

Phelan, V. (2020). *Overcoming: a memoir.* Dublin: Hachette Ireland.

Chapter 2

Brewis, J., Beck, V., Davies, A., & Matheson, J. (2017). *The Effects of Menopause Transition on Women's Economic Participation in the UK.* www.gov.uk. http://oro.open.ac.uk/59639/

Burden, L. (2021, June 18). *Millions of Women Exit Workforce for a Little-Talked About Reason.* Bloomberg Quint. https://www.bloomberg.com/news/articles/2021-06-18/women-are-leaving-the-workforce-for-a-little-talked-about-reason

Das, R. (2019, July 24). *Menopause Unveils Itself as The Next Big Opportunity In Femtech.* Forbes. https://www.forbes.com/sites/reenitadas/2019/07/24/menopause-unveils-itself-as-the-next-big-opportunity-in-femtech/

OlaOlorun, F. M., & Shen, W. (2020). Menopause. *Oxford Research Encyclopedia of Global Public Health.* https://doi.org/10.1093/acrefore/9780190632366.013.176

Panay, N., Anderson, R.A., Nappi, R.E., Vincent, A.J., Vujovic, S., Webber, L. and Wolfman, W. (2020). Premature ovarian insufficiency: an International Menopause Society White Paper. *Climacteric*, 23(5), pp.426–446.

Woods, N.F. and Mitchell, E.S. (2005). Symptoms during the perimenopause: prevalence, severity, trajectory, and significance in women's lives. *The American Journal of Medicine*, 118(12), pp.1405–1406.

Chapter 4

Carey, N. (2020). *Hacking the Code of Life: how gene editing will rewrite our futures.* London: Icon Books Ltd.

Channel 4. (2021). *Davina McCall: Sex, Myths, and the Menopause - All 4.* https://www.channel4.com/programmes/davina-mccall-sex-myths-and-the-menopause

Central Statistics Office. (2019). *Suicide Statistics - CSO - Central Statistics Office.* https://www.cso.ie/en/statistics/birthsdeathsandmarriages/suicidestatistics/

Central Statistics Office. (2019). *Population - CSO - Central Statistics Office.*; CSO. https://www.cso.ie/en/statistics/population/

Gates, M. (2020). *The Moment of Lift: how empowering women changes the world.* New York: Flatiron Books.

Jung, C. G., & Campbell, J. (1976). *The Portable Jung.* London: Penguin Books.

Lipton, B. H. (2016). *The Biology of Belief: unleashing the power of consciousness, matter & miracles.* California: Hay House.

National Women's Council of Ireland. (2018). *Out of Silence: Women's mental health in their own words.* Dublin: National Women's Council of Ireland. https://www.nwci.ie/images/uploads/NWCI_MentalHealth_Oct19_WEB.pdf

Perz, J. and Ussher, J.M. (2008). "The horror of this living decay": Women's negotiation and resistance of medical discourses around menopause and midlife. *Women's Studies International Forum*, 31(4), pp.293–299.

Robertson, I. (2021). *How Confidence Works: the new science of self -belief, why some people learn it and others don't.* London: Bantam Press.

Chapter 5

Ayers, B., Forshaw, M. and Hunter, M.S. (2010). The impact of attitudes towards the menopause on women's symptom experience: A systematic review. *Maturitas*, 65(1), pp.28–36.

Barlow, D.H. (2018). A long and winding road. *Menopause*, 25(12), pp.1395–1400.

Beck, V., Brewis, J. and Davies, A. (2018). The post-re/productive: researching the menopause. *Journal of Organizational Ethnography*, 7(3), pp.247–262.

Clark, J. H. (2007). A critique of Women's Health Initiative Studies (2002-2006). *Nuclear Receptor Signaling*, [online] 4. Available at: https://www.ncbi.nlm.nih.gov/pmc/articles/PMC1630688/ [Accessed 27 Apr. 2019].

Cleghorn, E. (2021). *Unwell women: a journey of medicine and myth in a man-made world.* London: Weidenfeld & Nicolson.

Criado Perez, C. (2019). *Invisible Women: exposing data bias in a world designed for men.* New York: Vintage.

de Salis, I., Owen-Smith, A., Donovan, J.L. and Lawlor, D.A. (2017). Experiencing menopause in the UK: The interrelated narratives of normality, distress, and transformation. *Journal of Women & Aging*, 30(6), pp.520–540.

Dillaway, H. (2015). Menopause: Deficiency Disease or Normal Reproductive Transition? In *The wrong prescription for women: how medicine and media create a "need" for treatments, drugs, and surgery.* California: Praeger.

Fyans, P. (2021). *The Invisible Job: parenting, running a home and dividing responsibility*. Dublin: Orpen Press.

Greer, G. (2018). *The Change: women, ageing and the menopause*. London: Bloomsbury Publishing.

Gunter, J. (2021). *The Menopause Manifesto: own your health with facts and feminism*. Ontario: Random House Canada.

Hollis, J. (2006). *Finding Meaning in the Second Half of Life: how to finally, really grow up*. New York: Gotham Books.

Mattern, S. P. (2021). *The Slow Moon Climbs: the science, history, and meaning of menopause*. New York: Princeton University Press.

Miller, L. (2021). *The Awakened Brain: the psychology of spirituality and our search for meaning*. London: Allen Lane.

Newhart, M.R. (2013). Menopause matters: The implications of menopause research for studies of midlife health. *Health Sociology Review*, 22(4), pp.365–376.

Northrup, C. (2021). *The Wisdom of Menopause : creating physical and emotional health during the change*. New York: Bantam Dell.

Sheehy, G. (1998). *The Silent Passage: menopause*. New York: Pocket Books.

Sieghart, M. A. (2021). *The Authority Gap*. London: Random House.

Steinke, D. (2020). *Flash Count Diary : a new story about the menopause*. Edinburgh: Canongate.

Voicu, I. (2018). The Social Construction of Menopause as disease: A literature review. *Journal of Comparative Research in Anthropology and Sociology*, 9(2), pp. 11–21.

WHO Scientific Group on Research on the Menopause & World Health Organization.(1981). Research on the menopause: report of a WHO scientific group [meeting held in Geneva from 8 to 12 December 1980]. In *apps.who.int*. World Health Organization. https://apps.who.int/iris/handle/10665/41526

Wilson, R. A. (1966). *Feminine Forever*. London: W.H. Allen.

Chapter 7

Central Statistics Office. (2019). *Suicide Statistics – CSO – Central Statistics Office*. https://www.cso.ie/en/statistics/birthsdeathsandmarriages/suicidestatistics/

Erikson, E. H., & Erikson, J. M. (1998). *The Life Cycle Completed*. New York: W.W. Norton.

McQuaide, S. (1998). Discontent at Midlife: Issues and Considerations in Working toward Women's Weil-Being. *Families in Society: The Journal of Contemporary Social Services*, 79(5), pp.532–542.

Northrup, C. (2021). *The Wisdom of Menopause: creating physical and emotional health during the change*. New York: Bantam Dell.

Pope, A., & Wurlitzer, S. H. (2017). *Wild Power*. California: Hay House.

Utz, R.L. (2011). Like mother, (not) like daughter: The social construction of menopause and aging. *Journal of Aging Studies*, 25(2), pp.143–154.

Chapter 8

Department of Health. (2020). *The Women's Health Taskforce*. https://www.gov.ie/en/campaigns/-womens-health/

Chapter 11

Baker, S. (2021). *The Shift: how I (lost and) found myself after 40 - and you can too.* London: Coronet.

Barlow, D.H. (2018). A long and winding road. *Menopause*, 25(12), pp.1395–1400.

Beck, V., Brewis, J. and Davies, A. (2018). The post-re/productive: researching the menopause. *Journal of Organizational Ethnography*, 7(3), pp.247–262.

Beck, V., Brewis, J., & Davies, A. (2019). The remains of the taboo: experiences, attitudes, and knowledge about menopause in the workplace. *Climacteric*, 23(2), pp. 158–164.

Brewis, J. (2020a). *Menopause awareness and higher education - guidance | Advance HE.* Www.advance-He.ac.uk. https://www.advance-he.ac.uk/knowledge-hub/menopause-awareness-and-higher-education-guidance

Brewis, J. (2020b). The health and socioeconomic impact on menopausal women of working from home. *Case Reports in Women's Health*, 27, p. e00229.

Candito, M. (2019). *Ignite Your Feminine Power: inspiration to rise up and change the world.* (n.p).

Hickey, M., Szabo, R.A. and Hunter, M.S. (2017). Non-hormonal treatments for menopausal symptoms. *BMJ*, 359, p.j5101.

Hunter, M., & Smith, M. (2021). *Managing hot flushes and night sweats: a cognitive behavioural self-help guide to the menopause.* Abingdon: Routledge.

Krajewski, S. (2018b). Advertising menopause: you have been framed. *Continuum*, 33(1), pp. 137–148.

Ussher, J. M. (2010). Are We Medicalizing Women's Misery? A Critical Review of Women's Higher Rates of Reported Depression. *Feminism & Psychology*, 20(1), pp. 9–35.

Ussher, J. M. (2011). *The Madness of Women: myth and experience.* Abingdon: Routledge.

Chapter 12

Baker, F. C., Willoughby, A. R., Sassoon, S. A., Colrain, I. M., & de Zambotti, M. (2015). Insomnia in women approaching menopause: Beyond perception. *Psychoneuroendocrinology*, 60, pp. 96–104.

Hickey, M., Szabo, R. A., & Hunter, M. S. (2017). Non-hormonal treatments for menopausal symptoms. *BMJ*, 359, p. j5101.

National European Healthcare Quality Reporting System. (NHQRS) (2019). *Statistics on Benzodiazepine prescribing in Ireland.* Dublin: Department of Health.

Prague, J., Roberts, R., Comninos, A., Clarke, S., Jayasena, C., Nash, Z., Doyle, C., Papadopoulou, D., Bloom, S., Mohideen, P., Panay, N., Hunter, M., Veldhuis, J., Webber, L., Huson, L., & Dhillo, W. (2017). Neurokinin 3 receptor antagonism as a novel treatment for menopausal hot flushes: a phase 2, randomised, double-blind, placebo-controlled trial. *Endocrine Abstracts*, 389(10081), pp. 1809–1820.

Rance, N. E., Dacks, P. A., Mittelman-Smith, M. A., Romanovsky, A. A., & Krajewski-Hall, S. J. (2013). Modulation of body temperature and LH secretion by hypothalamic KNDy (kisspeptin, neurokinin B and dynorphin) neurons: A novel hypothesis on the mechanism of hot flushes. *Frontiers in Neuroendocrinology*, 34(3), pp. 211–227.

Chapter 15

Baker, S. (2021). *The Shift : how I (lost and) found myself after 40 - and you can too.* London: Coronet.

Bates, L. (2016). *Everyday Sexism*. New York: Thomas Dunne Books, St. Martin's Griffin.

Boutcher, Y. N., Boutcher, S. H., Yoo, H. Y., & Meerkin, J. D. (2019). The Effect of Sprint Interval Training on Body Composition of Postmenopausal Women. *Medicine & Science in Sports & Exercise*, 51(7), pp. 1413–1419.

Chemaly, S. L. (2019). *Rage Becomes Her: the power of women's anger*. New York: Atria Books.

Krajewski, S. (2018a). Advertising menopause: you have been framed. *Continuum*, 33(1), pp. 137–148.

Krajewski, S. (2018b). Killer Whales and Killer Women: Exploring Menopause as a "Satellite Taboo" that Orbits Madness and Old Age. *Sexuality & Culture*, 23(2), pp. 605–620.

Steinke, D. (2020). *Flash Count Diary: a new story about the menopause*. Edinburgh: Canongate.

Chapter 17

Davie, G. (2007). From Believing without Belonging to Vicarious Religion: Understanding the Patterns of Religion in Modern Europe. In B. Pollack & D. V. A. Olson (Eds.), *The Role of Religion in Modern Societies*. Abingdon: Routledge.

Gottfried, S. (2014). *The Hormone Cure: reclaim balance, sleep, and sex drive; lose weight, feel focused, vital, and energized naturally with the Gottfried Protocol*. New York: Scribner.

Chapter 18

Delgado, D. (2017). *I Choose Joy: The Daily Gratitude Practice That Will Transform Your Life*. (n.p).

Merzenich, M. M. (2004). *Growing evidence of brain plasticity.* TED Conferences LLC. https://www.ted.com/talks/michael_merzenich_growing_evidence_of_brain_plasticity

Merzenich, M. M. (2013). *Soft-wired: how the new science of brain plasticity can change your life.* California: Parnassus Publishing, Ltd.

Chapter 20

Dillaway, H. E. (2012). Reproductive history as social context. Exploring how women talk about menopause and sexuality at midlife. In L. M. Carpenter & J. De Lamater (Eds.), *Sex for life: From virginity to Viagra, how sexuality changes throughout our lives.* New York: New York University Press.

Jack, G., Riach, K., Bariola, E., Pitts, M., Schapper, J., & Sarrel, P. (2016). Menopause in the workplace: What employers should be doing. *Maturitas*, 85, pp. 88–95.

McGowan, J. A., & Pottern, L. (2000). Commentary on the Women's Health Initiative. *Maturitas*, 34(2), pp. 109–112.

Further Reading

Books

Baker, S. (2021). *The Shift: how I (lost and) found myself after 40 - and you can too*. London: Coronet.

Barry, H. (2021). *Embracing Change: How to build resilience & make change work for you*. London: Orion Spring.

Beard, M. (2017). *Women & Power: a manifesto*. London: Liveright Publishing Corporation.

Brennan, S. (2021). *Beating Brain Fog: Your 30 Day Plan to Think Faster Sharper Better*. London: Orion Spring.

Chemaly, S. L. (2019). *Rage Becomes Her: the power of women's anger*. New York: Atria Books.

Cleghorn, E. (2021). *Unwell Women: a journey of medicine and myth in a man-made world*. London: Weidenfeld & Nicolson.

Criado Perez, C. (2020). *Invisible Women: exposing data bias in a world designed for men*. New York: Vintage.

Doyle, G. (2020). *Untamed*. New York: The Dial Press.

Fyans, P. (2021). *The Invisible Job: parenting, running a home and dividing responsibility*. Dublin: Orpen Press.

Greer, G. (2018). *The Change: women, ageing and the menopause*. London: Bloomsbury Publishing.

Hill, M. (2021). *Perimenopause Power: from hormone hell to harmony.* London: Green Tree.

Lesser, E. (2020). *Cassandra Speaks: when women are the storytellers, the human story changes.* New Wave: Harper Wave.

Mathews, M. (2020). *New Hot: taking on the menopause with attitude and style.* London: Vermilion.

Robertson, I. (2021). *How Confidence Works: the new science of self-belief, why some people learn it and others don't.* London: Penguin.

Scott, L. (2020). *The Double X Economy: the epic potential of empowering women.* London: Faber & Faber.

Sheehy, G. (1998). *The Silent Passage: menopause.* New York: Pocket Books.

Sieghart, M. A. (2021). *The Authority Gap.* London: Random House.

Stewart, M., & Wolloch, E. (2020). *Manage Your Menopause Naturally: the six-week guide to calming hot flashes & night sweats, getting your sex drive back, sharpening memory & reclaiming well-being.* San Francisco: New World Library.

Williams, N. (2017). *It's not you, it's your hormones: The essential guide for women over 40 to fight fat, fatigue and hormone havoc.* London: Practical Inspiration Publishing.

Wurlitzer, S. H. and Pope. A. (2017). *Wild Power.* California: Hay House.

Websites

Diane Danzebrink	www.dianedanzebrink.com/menopause
Dr Betsy Greenleaf	www.drbetsygreenleaf.com
Dr Easkey Britton	www.easkeybritton.com
Dr Louise Newson	www.menopausedoctor.co.uk
Dr Mark Rowe	www.drmarkrowe.com
Dr Mary Ryan	www.drmaryryan.com
Evolving Wisdom	www.evolvingwisdom.com
Global menopause	www.dignifiedmenopause.org
Health Talk	www.healthtalk.org/menopause
Ilona Madden	www.rightfood4u.ie
Irish Eco therapist Shirley Gleeson	www. ecowellnessconsulting.com
Jojo Bailey/Gray area drinking	www.jojobailey.com
Katharine Gale	www.Fluxstate.co.uk
Lorna Ivo	www.perimenopost.com
Lorraine Boyce	www.downbelowphysio.ie
Marie Keating Foundation	www.mariekeating.ie
Meg Mathews	www.megmathewsmenopause.com
Midlife Women Rock Project	www.midlifewomenrockproject.com
Nicki Williams	www.happyhormonesforlife.com

Rely _on Stella App	www.onstella.com
Roisin Nic Chleirigh	www.confidentwomenireland.ie
Sally Anne Brady	www.theirishmenopause.ie
The British Menopause Society	www.thebms.org.uk
The Daisy Network	www.daisynetwork.com
The Health service Executive (HSE)	www.HSE.ie/menopause
The Mac Study Trinity College Dublin	www.macstudy.ie
The Menopause Hub	www.menopausehub.ie
The Science of a Meaningful Life	www.greatergood.berkeley.edu

Campaigns

#100DaysOfWalking Dr Ciara Kelly's campaign which starts in January each year on social media

#MakeMenopauseMatter campaign in the UK

#TheIrishMenopauseMission in Ireland

ACKNOWLEDGEMENTS

The journey towards writing this book began in 2018. I have to sincerely thank Dr Jacinta Byrne-Doran, my academic supervisor who suggested I review the research on midlife women, which she mentioned were an understudied cohort in academia. To Dr Mary Benson, Maynooth University, who enabled me to see the power of story in interviewing and researching women's lives.

To everyone at *Social Entrepreneurs Ireland*. Mentors, guides, and the super peer-to-peer support groups, I thank you. You have been hugely instrumental in assisting me in moving forward with the project which is now becoming a book. I have been very fortunate to have you all along the way.

I owe a great debt of gratitude to all involved in social enterprise in Waterford for helping me realise the idea about the cafés. Liz Riches, Nicola Kent, Michael Kelly *GIY Ireland*, Local Enterprise Office (LEO) Waterford, and Tammy Darcy from *The Shona Project*, a super mentor when I started out. To all at *Waterford Health Park* who invited us to run the *Midlife Women Rock Cafés* monthly from the beautiful and comfortable surroundings of the atrium, a huge thank you.

To the women who attended the cafés in the early months. You believed in what I was doing as you returned again and again. For that, I will be forever grateful. Special mention to Susan, Elaine, Ger, Sinead, Helen, Ruth, Anna, Jennifer, Gabrielle, and Barbara.

A huge thank you to Nuala Browne, at *Meraki Marketing* for teaching me all that I now know about social media. One is never too old to learn. Thanks, must also go to Roisin Nic Chlerigh who has been a super support and advocate for menopause on her Kilkenny community radio show.

There are so many to thank over this past year Dr Joanna Martin, Sara Price, Karen Skidmore, Kate Wolf, Helen Connolly and the many awesomely wonderful women I have been privileged to get to know through the One *of Many* community. A sincere and huge thank you to the early readers of the proposal and manuscript Claire, Morag, Nicola, Patty. I would not have made it here without your constructive feedback and encouragement. It enabled me to keep going and to Anita for our monthly motivational zoom calls. Fiona Lafferty I thank you for believing in me when this book was only an idea, your generosity of time and expertise in early edits helped me to keep moving forward.

To my Monday and Thursday night tennis gangs. I often say to my children, "An hour on a tennis court is like an hour's therapy with the added bonus of losing some calories and having some laughs." Thank you for your warm friendship and ongoing support. You all rock.

A special thanks has to go to my dear friend and fabulous Mum of two, Marian O'Nuallain. You have been on this journey from the very beginning, and a tremendous support. I am sure there were times you thought I was really losing my mind as I persisted with the advocacy around menopause.

To the truly amazing nursing group of '86 who enabled and encouraged me to start this enquiry into menopause. I wholeheartedly thank you for your constant friendship and continuous support over the past 35 years. Looking forward to February and our annual reunion already.

I have to mention my close extended family, my wonderful aunts, uncles, and cousins who have all been hugely influential in my life growing up in Kerry. You know who you are. My two brothers John and Michael, and sisters Tess, Eils, Angie, and families. Let's continue the sea swimming. My Mom, Mary Ellen, and Dad, Michael RIP, for whom family was always first.

To Geraldine Walsh my editor and proof-reader. You have been amazing. You made the process easy. To Orla Kelly publisher extraordinaire, you worked your magic, and I am so grateful with the end result. I really love it.

To the many wonderful women whom I have met on their menopause journeys and to those who have given of their time to be interviewed. This book would not exist only for you, for this I sincerely thank you.

Finally, to my partner in life for 28 years my husband John. Thank you for your patience and ongoing support in getting this book to the finish line. We are blessed to be parents to John, Laura, Aly, and Will, who have lit up our lives in so many ways. Thank you Four, for your encouragement, WhatsApp messages, memes, and hugs as I completed this book. So proud of you all and truly grateful for your love and support.

Connect with Breeda

Breeda is available to do podcast guesting workplace presentations and is a Keynote speaker. In addition to running free events, Breeda also offers private consultations, courses and workplace packages. To work with Breeda or find out more, go to midlifewomenrockproject.com.

Please Review

Dear reader,

If you enjoyed this book, I would really appreciate if you could leave a review on Amazon or Goodreads. Your opinion counts and it does influence buyer decisions on whether to purchase the book or not. Reviews can also open doors to new and bigger audiences for the author and helps get this book into the hands of those who most need to hear its message.

Printed in Great Britain
by Amazon

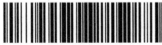